RUNNING TO KEEP FIT

Brian Mitchell is a British Amateur Athletic Board senior coach, with more than twenty years of coaching experience. He has been an active runner since his schooldays, still runs at least four times a week, and as a teacher is very closely involved with school and club athletes of all abilities.

He has written four books on running and athletics, is the author of numerous articles published in British and American journals, and is a regular contributor to *Athletics Weekly*.

TEACH YOURSELF BOOKS

RUNNING TO KEEP FIT

Brian Mitchell

TEACH YOURSELF BOOKS

Hodder and Stoughton

First edition 1980
Second edition 1984

British Library Cataloguing in Publication Data

Mitchell, Brian, *1930*
Running to keep fit—2nd ed—(Teach yourself books)
1. Running—Physiological aspects
2. Physical fitness
I. Title
613.7'1   GV1061

ISBN 0 340 34667 1

Printed and bound in Great Britain
for Hodder and Stoughton Educational,
a division of Hodder and Stoughton Ltd,
Mill Road, Dunton Greeen, Sevenoaks, Kent,
by Richard Clay (The Chaucer Press) Ltd, Bungay, Suffolk

Contents

Introduction

Most people can run. Therefore most people could have the physical fitness that running creates. It is the purpose of this book to look at the simple act of running, how it may be used and pursued through the early stages of 'jogging' to the point where it offers quite a high level of fitness, yet remains something which a man or woman of almost any age, or in any circumstance, can achieve. There is plenty of evidence from all parts of the world that running need not be the possession of an élite few.

In these pages, all aspects of running for fitness are examined and it has been presumed that the reader starts with just a flicker of intention; that he or she is interested enough to consider non-competitive exercise and to test the truth of what is explained.

There is nothing complicated or difficult (or expensive!) about starting to run or about progressing to fitness. The principles upon which 'fitness running' is based are those of athletics and exercise physiology. They are well established and easily grasped. They centre on the idea of a particular degree and balance of stress and recovery; the idea can be put into immediate practice by anyone and will operate for the individual. The help offered here is meant to be direct and practical: what to do and how to do it, with a glance at why.

Fitness and health are enjoyable. Fitness is most easily created by running, which is itself enjoyable. Of course, running is not the only means of achieving fitness, but it is the most practicable, and the most far reaching.

B.M.

I

A State of Mind

Look to your health; and if you have it, praise
God, and value it next to a good conscience.

Izaak Walton

The person who is looking for physical fitness is, most probably, someone who is aware of its absence. Various motives
prompt us to take exercise, in competitive sport or apart from
it. Most sports create and demand a noticeable level of fitness,
but this fitness is a by-product or necessary possession rather
than the main aim of the sportsman. Even the competitive
boxer, runner, cyclist, will develop fitness because it allows
him to function successfully, not just because it is something
he wants for itself; it will be enjoyed when it is acquired, and
might become a predominant goal, but usually it is not the
overriding factor in training. In the young, particularly,
motives which prompt participation in sport are probably the
development of skill, belonging to a team or club, pleasure in
winning, enjoyment of physical movement. When you are
young, you do not have to worry much about fitness. When
you are no longer young, and when you live in a so-called
'advanced' society, which does not encourage or enhance
physical fitness, you may become strongly aware of your own
lack of fitness. Perhaps a friend or colleague suffers a heart-
attack, perhaps you merely find that you cannot tackle a game
or a holiday walk as you once could. By some means, awareness
of your condition grows.

It is in this state of mind, provoked by a state of body, that you may begin positively to look for a way of getting, and keeping, fit. What is argued in this book is relevant to young and old, men and women, but it will have particular meaning for the person who is already looking for fitness and for a simple, effective way of reaching that enviable state.

Before examining the process and the product, the 'stab at longevity', as one elderly runner called it, it might help if the meaning of the word 'fit' were established, since it is one of the two upon which this book hinges.

If something 'fits', it takes its rightful place without undue difficulty. If food is 'fit' for human consumption, it can go inside us and do its job of nourishing. If a man is 'fit' for walking, or golf, or climbing a mountain, he is able to do those things and not suffer for it. If he is 'fit' to drive to work, sit at a desk all day, drive home and sit in front of the television all evening, he may be said to be 'fit' to take his place in one part of modern society. This last example reveals the irony of being 'fit' for that circumstance which will itself limit 'fitness'. To be 'fit' for sitting in a chair is not a guarantee for being 'fit' to dig the garden or stay alive beyond fifty. The 'fitness' of a young person (so tenuous and so quickly lost or foolishly abused) is enviable, even beautiful, and therefore essentially right – or 'fit' – for men, women and animals. It is this kind of 'fitness', the proper inheritance, the physical perfection, the immaculate functioning, to which the word should refer. If neglect, or fashion, work against such 'fitness', and physical activity restores it, then the argument on behalf of running to keep fit is strong. Running does keep you fit. It keeps you fit to meet demands which the body should be able to meet – certainly a round of golf, a long walk, a game in the garden and a desire to take part in these activities. Above all, it keeps you fit to enjoy life, to allow you to take your rightful place without difficulty amongst those activities which appeal to you, and for which you need a capable physical mechanism (yourself!).

In a state of mind which is turning, however tentatively, towards fitness and running, then, consider what attracts and what deflects.

The main attraction is the knowledge that running could

take almost anyone from an unnecessarily poor physical condition to an acceptable condition, that the destination is attractive, the journey more-or-less free, and the pleasure and satisfaction utterly private. Pride is involved, and a special kind of release which is found in action, movement and intention; these are positive factors, which do lead somewhere and do offer, also, their own intrinsic rewards. In our society, they imply a certain degree of opposition to current attitudes and behaviour, but that could be good, if those attitudes are leading towards ill health.

A kind of fear is what deflects and dissuades. This may, for example, be fear of doing physical damage to oneself, or just fear of the supposed discomfort involved in running, or of possible failure, or the trivial mockery sometimes thrown at the runner on the public highway. None of these fears need prohibit. A medical examination should precede new or unusual activity, and once there is clearance to start, no chronic weaknesses identified, you can be sure that the fitness running (if rightly pursued and cajoled) will do good, not harm. Discomfort is avoided as a policy, and the practical applications of this are explained later in the book; essentially, you build from a tolerable level and progress to another tolerable level, and so on, with undue discomfort as a sign to be acknowledged. Failure need not be entertained, because each person is merely proceeding month by month either to reach or to maintain an individual level of fitness. Since there will be no rigid target and no absolute criterion, there will be no failure. This is not to say that, assessing your own capacity against somebody else's, you might not feel small, but that is a motive for continuing. As for mockery, in Britain at least, it is part of the runner's life to be chanted at by idiot bystanders, it does no harm and you are free to shout back if you wish. The runner need not doubt himself in these circumstances.

Knowing that fitness may be had, that we can be responsible for our own state, unless we are struck by sheer misfortune, it is helpful to consider the notion of a plan.

It is helpful to look positively in the direction of physical fitness, rather than towards hospitals and doctors, seeing fitness as something better than an absence of disease, conceiving a commitment to the accomplishment of fitness. The words of the historian, R. H. Tawney, are persuasive:

'For the purpose is, in the first place, a principle of limitation. It determines the end for which, and therefore the limits within which, an activity is to be carried on. It divides what is worth doing from what is not, and settles the scale upon which what is worth doing ought to be done. It is, in the second place, a principle of unity, because it supplies a common end to which efforts can be directed . . . It is, in the third place, a principle of apportionment or distribution.'

The practice of limitation and apportionment in running training is looked at in chapters four and five; it is enough here to note that the state of mind of the potential runner embraces 'purpose' and, therefore, plan. The plan does not have to be subtle or detailed, but rather the sort of outline plan you might make in the winter for a summer holiday. This is a draught plan really, probably not even written down, indicating a purpose, persuading yourself that you do intend to run for fitness and to find a means within the context of your daily life. It will indicate what is to be done, when and where.

It will be said, though it ought not to be, that the busy citizen cannot find time for regular exercise, just as it is said that he, or she, cannot find time for reading, or making music, or growing food, or any of the thousands of interesting and enjoyable activities available to intelligent mankind. To claim that there is not time for physical exercise is like claiming that there is not time to eat properly. There has to be. The example of the competitive athlete is one to be followed here. In Britain, and in many other countries to a greater or lesser degree, there are capable athletes who train daily, and even twice daily, sometimes alongside demanding jobs, families and homes. Since the fitness runner is only going to do a minute fraction of the running/exercise carried out by the competitive athlete, and since the rewards are so seriously worth having, the state of mind which says there is not time is really a state of mind to be changed by reason and judgement. The purpose – fitness – is enough to bring down this particular road-block. We all have twenty-four hours in our day. The practical question is: within our own limitations, what can be done?

The special frame of mind of the woman runner, or potential runner, must be considered, too, because ridiculously enough, it remains more difficult, even in progressive societies, for a woman to take up running. Again, the complete obstacle is sent crashing to the ground by the examples of what has been done by women, particularly in the USA and Europe. A strong, independent mind is needed, but there are plenty of female ones about! Women can do all that men can do in this sphere, even if a little less swiftly. The final of the women's 800 metres at the Montreal Olympics proved that, with seven athletes doing inside two minutes and racing as forcefully as ever any man did. Perhaps the best example and proof that women need not hesitate, is that of Katherine Switzer, an American who barged into the 1967 Boston Marathon race, at a time when women were not allowed to take part. She said, 'I understood it to be an open race, which as far as I was concerned included me.' Later, she pointed out that the central question affecting women runners is, Why can't I do what I want to do? It has become clear since the 1960s that women can do the running they want to do, to race or to keep fit; they have fought for this and gained the freedom of mind and action, though it is still not theirs, of course, in many parts of the world. If a woman wants to be fit and trim, and to be so by means of the running she enjoys, she can and will. Authorities who sought to control the adult woman's competitive distance have now relented and only the younger runner is now, sensibly, restricted. But there is no authority, luckily, in fitness running, other than that of individual desire and conscience. And the physical differences, which are limitations in competitive athletics, do not affect at all the principles or availability of preparation and progress. These are the same for women as for men in fitness running.

To summarise the state of mind of the potential fitness runner, it may be said to be that of someone who has been prompted to action, wants to act and may have slight doubts about the practicability. But the process and the goal are enjoyable, helpful, valuable. The obstacles can be crossed. What is to be gained is physical fitness, the means by which we live at all.

2

The Physiological Effects of Regular Running

J. L. Mayhew, Ph.D. (Northeast Missouri
State University), and W. F. Riner, Jr., Ph.D.
(University of South Carolina)

Perhaps no other activity has been so widely studied by exercise scientists as running. Individuals from six to sixty years old have been the focal points of numerous investigations into the physiological effects of running. In almost all of these studies, running has proven to have positive benefits on the health and fitness of the subjects, the degree often depending on the intensity, duration and frequency of the training sessions.

The growing interest in jogging and running has prompted even greater scrutiny by physicians, exercise physiologists and coaches. With new, more sophisticated techniques, exercise scientists are continuing to discover valuable information concerning the acute and chronic effects of running on the body. Our purpose here is to review some of the findings and provide insight into their meaning.

At the outset it might be wise to distinguish between 'jogging' and 'running'. From the standpoint of energetics, man usually chooses to change from walking to running at a speed of about 80 metres/minute (8 km/hr). It is at this point that it requires less energy to run slowly than to walk fast. Some experts feel that 'jogging' involves speed up to 5 : 20 per kilometre. Any speed faster than 5 : 20 per kilometre is considered 'running'. Beyond these points the difference appears to be as much semantic as real. Needless to say, whether you jog or run, the physiological rewards of individually tailored exercise programmes can be as great for the jogger as for the Olympian.

For our purposes, we will call running any locomotion in which both feet lose contact with the ground during the stride. More important than arguments over the name of the activity are the biochemical and physiological changes that occur when one participates in running for an extended period.

Cardiorespiratory changes

In perhaps no other system of the body are the effects of running as profound as in the cardiorespiratory (C–R) system. The C–R system includes the heart and its blood vessels (the pulmonary arteries). These two seemingly different organs work so closely to supply oxygen to working muscles that they are actually considered as a functional unit.

The heart
The heart is made up of four chambers. The top two chambers (the atria) serve to fill the bottom two chambers (the ventricles). Actually, the atria are not very important during rest, but may function to aid ventricular filling during the high heart rates of exercise. The ventricles pump blood to the lungs and the body simultaneously. The right ventricle pumps blood to the lungs where it takes on a fresh supply of oxygen. Upon returning to the heart, the oxygen-rich blood is pumped to the remainder of the body by the left ventricle.

When the pumping work of the heart is increased, the cardiac muscle responds by growing in size (hypertrophy). If the increased work of the heart is caused by pushing against an elevated blood pressure, the cardiac hypertrophy is pathological and may result in severe medical problems for the victim. However, if the increased work of the heart is to pump greater volumes of blood to working muscles, the heart enlarges in order to achieve this task more efficiently. This is often termed the 'athletic heart' and is mislabelled as pathological. It is, in fact, a normal response to endurance training and provides a stronger, more efficient heart.

In almost all individuals who engage in endurance running, the growth of the heart is due to enlargement of the ventricular chambers. These enlarged chambers mean that a person will have a greater stroke/volume (quantity of blood ejected with each contraction of the heart). As a result of a regular endurance training programme, the left ventricle, which pumps blood to the working muscles, expands to the greatest degree.

In addition to the larger size of the ventricles, the force with which they contract is increased with training. The ventricles, therefore, empty to a greater extent with each heart beat. The results of the greater ventricular volume and the stronger contraction provide the endurance-trained person with the larger stroke-volume.

The greater pumping capacity of the heart means that less work need be done by that organ to supply the body with oxygen-laden blood. Thus, one of the most obvious changes resulting from a training programme is a reduction in the resting and exercise heart rates. While sitting quietly the trained individual will notice that the resting heart rate has been reduced 5–15 beats/minute. Instead of the normal rate of 60–80 beats/minute, his heart may beat as few as 40–55 times each minute.

If this individual began running easily for several miles, taking the pulse rate at the conclusion, he or she might note a similar reduction in rate. The heart is under less stress to accomplish the same amount of exercise as before training. If the individual improves the resting heart rate from 70 to 60 beats/minute through training, the person will save approximately 14,000 beats a day or about five million heart beats a year! Since the only rest the heart gets is between contractions, this 14 per cent improvement in efficiency means less work for the heart.

The lungs

The lungs are made up of millions of tiny air sacs (called alveoli) at the terminal ends of the air passages. These alveoli provide about 70–90 square metres of surface area from which oxygen is absorbed by the blood. The size of one's lungs is largely dependent on the body size and training appears to have little effect on lung size. Fortunately, however, lung size does not limit one's capacity or performance.

During quiet breathing the diaphragm is the principal muscle of inspiration. Expiration is a passive process with the recoil of the ribs doing the major part of the work. At various levels of exercise, however, both inspiration and expiration are active processes. The muscles between the ribs (the inter-costals) become more active in lifting and lowering the rib cage to bring air into the lungs; the diaphragm continues to operate during inhalation and the abdominal muscles aid in expiration during heavy exercise. It is these muscles that often become sore when an individual exercises for the first time or trains (or races) harder than he or she is accustomed to.

Some exercising individuals have been bothered by a 'stitch', a pain in the side usually at the border of the lower ribs on either side. This is usually due to lack of sufficient blood flow to the diaphragm. In unfit persons it is probably due to the unaccustomed strenuousness of exercise breathing. It may happen, however, in fit subjects and is then likely to be due to inadequate or improper warm-up, or undigested stomach contents restricting the fall of the diaphragm. Many tech-niques have been advocated for relief from this problem, none of which appears to have a sound scientific basis. Perhaps the best advice is to eat no later than two–three hours before exercising, warm-up well before beginning hard exercise, and maintain running rhythm as close to normal as possible to avoid unusual twisting on the trunk, another factor thought to contribute to a stitch.

As a result of endurance training several changes take place in lung function. Three of the most important are increased perfusion rate, greater diffusion capacity and improved ventilatory efficiency. With the greater amount of blood pumped from the heart, dormant capillaries (microscopic blood vessels) in the lungs are perfused with blood. This enhances the diffusion of oxygen from the lungs into the blood, a phenomenon known as diffusion capacity. Following training there may be a two- to three-fold increase in the diffusion rate of oxygen into the blood. This is important since at the higher heart rates of exercise blood courses through the pulmonary arteries rapidly. The greater diffusion rate aids in the complete saturation of the blood with oxygen.

As fitness is acquired, efficiency of ventilating the lungs improves. Indeed, much of the feeling of 'being in shape' is due to the reduced respiratory distress during exercise. Once fitness is acquired, less lung ventilation is required per unit of oxygen absorbed by the body. In other words, you are required to breathe smaller volumes of air into the lungs in order to meet the body's oxygen requirement. This usually means fewer breaths are taken per minute, lessening the stress on the respiratory muscles to ventilate the lungs.

Sometimes a form of respiratory distress relief occurs momentarily during a hard exercise session and is called 'second wind'. Although the exact physiological basis for this phenomenon is not fully understood, a relief in the breathing process is one of the most often mentioned factors. Second wind is not confined to the beginning exerciser; it may occur at any level of fitness and at any time during an exercise session. It may occur in the easiest of training sessions and bypass you during the toughest sessions or vice versa.

Many runners have asked if there is a 'best' pattern for breathing while running. Should one breathe through the nose or the mouth? Although most runners report breathing in a rhythm with their strides (breathing in on two strides and out on two strides), the best way is the most comfortable way for each individual. There are many patterns which result in breathing frequencies between 30 and 50 times per minute for runners exercising at the same pace. As for the passage of air into the lungs, breathing through the nose and mouth provides the maximum amount of air flow. There is no danger of freezing the lungs in cold weather since the air is warmed and moistened by the time it reaches the voice box. Again, the pattern of breathing is an individual matter and the most comfortable pattern for you is the 'best' one.

Blood changes

The blood is made up of two parts. The first part, the plasma or fluid part, serves to transport the second part, the cells. In the normal individual a small blood sample drawn from the fingertip can be spun for several minutes to reveal this separation. The heavier cells settle to the bottom of the test–tube while the fluid plasma remains at the top. This is termed the haematocrit and reveals the percentage of your blood that is cells. Most of these cells are red blood cells (RBC) which carry the oxygen-transporting compound haemoglobin. Haemoglobin is a protein-iron complex which binds oxygen at the lungs and delivers it to the cells.

Many runners have been disturbed by reports that chronic exercise may cause them to become anaemic. Anaemia is that condition caused by a deficiency of red blood cells and/or haemoglobin. The simple clinical tests for haemoglobin or haematocrit may indeed show the athlete to be apparently anaemic. In point of fact, the chronic exerciser may have the condition known as 'athletic' or 'pseudo-anaemia'. Because the clinical tests are based on a per 100 millilitre standard of blood unit, the greater increase in plasma volume experienced by most runners will, in effect, dilute the cell volume. In actuality, the individual engaged in long-term endurance exercise may develop a 20 per cent greater blood volume and haemoglobin content than the untrained counterpart. Since it is total haemoglobin that counts in the oxygen-carrying capacity of the blood, the trained individual need not be alarmed at somewhat lower values on the clinical tests.

To combat this apparent anaemia, however, many runners take iron or folic acid pills. Research by a British team has shown that there is no difference in the haemoglobin or red blood cell content between athletes taking these supplements and athletes not taking these additives. Dutch physiologists note that while the diet of most training individuals is sufficient in iron content, excessive fat intake may hinder the absorption of that iron by the intestines. This is yet another good reason for the exercising person to minimise dietary fat intake.

Haematuria

The acute effect of strenuous running on blood components may at times alarm some participants. Although it is not particularly common, the urine may sometimes be stained pink or reddish in the hours after a hard run or race. This is most likely due to the removal by the kidneys of the components of broken blood cells and damaged muscle fibres. Although the complete scientific explanation of this phenomenon is not known, some experts suspect that it may be related to the hardness of the running surface and/or the stress of the exercise. While running on hard surfaces, such as paved roads and sidewalks, blood cells passing through the feet may be ruptured by the concussion spilling their haemoglobin into the blood. During strenuous exercise some of the muscle fibres may be damaged allowing myoglobin (a substance much like haemoglobin that carries oxygen in the muscles) to filter into the blood. The kidneys do an excellent job of removing these residues, sometimes to the consternation of the runner. The condition is temporary in almost all cases, and there is usually no damage to the body. The use of well-padded training shoes may all but eliminate the problem.

Blood lipids

With regard to coronary heart disease much attention has been given to the effect that regular running has on the way blood carries fats (lipids). One of the blood lipids receiving the most attention in the past was cholesterol. A high level of cholesterol was generally identified as a coronary heart disease risk factor, increasing the chances of developing the disease. Often those individuals found to have high cholesterol values are placed on restricted diets and medication to reduce the cholesterol level and their chances of developing heart disease. Women, while having almost as high blood cholesterol levels as men, were thought to be protected from heart disease by the 'female hormones'.

Recent research has revealed that it is not so much the total amount of cholesterol in the blood, although that may still be of concern, but how it is carried that matters. Cholesterol may be carried by lipoproteins, substances that bind with the cholesterol to transport it through the blood. When cholesterol binds with low-density lipoproteins (LDL) it is easily given up to be stored in the vessel walls, leading to the disease atherosclerosis.

This disease is a progressive deposition of lipids in the vessel walls causing a reduced diameter and restricted blood flow. The chances of developing a clot (thrombus) in one of the affected arteries is greatly increased. The most likely place for this to happen is in the coronary arteries and the result is a myocardial infarction ('heart-attack').

When cholesterol is carried by high-density lipoprotein (HDL), however, it is not so readily given up to storage but may instead be transported to the liver for breakdown, conversion to glucose or excretion. Thus many authorities are supporting high HDL levels as offering protection against coronary heart disease. It is now known that women generally have higher levels of HDL than men, which may be the key factor affording them greater protection against heart disease.

How does all this affect the exercising individual? Careful testing of élite distance runners has shown their HDL levels to be far above and their LDL levels far below age-matched non-exercising individuals. Furthermore, some studies have noted an increase in HDL with strenuous exercise. It is likely that a regular running programme improves the way your blood handles fats. Whether this factor alone provides protection against coronary heart disease remains to be seen. While it is not likely that high HDL would be the only factor of protection, the other conditions accompanying an exercise programme, *viz.*, lowered blood pressure, moderation of diet, adequate rest, reduced tension, and physiological efficiency, would greatly reduce the likelihood of you developing heart disease.

Oxygen intake changes

Closely paralleling the change in C–R function resulting from exercise is the ability of the working muscle cells to supply energy. As long as the demand for energy does not exceed the supply, an exercise can be carried on for an extended period. The key to the entire process is the rate at which the working cells can take up and use oxygen to supply the needed energy. If the exercise is such that the demand does not exceed the supply, it is termed 'aerobic'. This word literally means 'in the presence of oxygen' and refers to the complex biochemical processes by which the cell produces energy.

This energy production takes place inside each muscle cell within specialised structures called mitochondria. All of the biochemical enzymes necessary for aerobic energy production are located within these tiny structures where they serve to release the energy locked in nutrient molecules by carrying their atomic electrons ultimately to oxygen. The greater the individual's capacity to take in and utilise oxygen along this metabolic pathway, the greater the capability for energy production. Therefore, the maximal rate at which a person can take in oxygen (maximal oxygen intake or VO_2max) has gained wide acceptance as the best measure of one's physical fitness.

When the demand for oxygen exceeds the ability of the respiratory enzymes of the mitochondria to supply it, energy must be derived from 'anaerobic' sources, those that occur without oxygen being present. This is a short-term venture, unfortunately, since the end result of anaerobic metabolism is lactic acid. A build-up of lactic acid in the muscles may be one of the prime causes of fatigue, making you slow down or stop for recovery.

One of the primary objectives of running training, therefore, is to increase the capacity which respiratory enzymes have for delivering oxygen along the biochemical chain. Several studies on animals and man have noted as much as a two-fold increase in these enzymes with running training. This phenomenon allows the cell to produce more energy aerobically, forestalling the transition to anaerobic metabolism and the rise in lactic acid.

Much attention has recently been given to the anaerobic threshold, that point on the energy continuum at which excess lactic acid begins to appear in the blood. In the untrained person this occurs at about 50 per cent of the VO_2max. In the moderately trained individual this point may be 65–70 per cent of VO_2max, while in the highly trained endurance athlete it may be as high as 90 per cent of VO_2 max. The improvement in the anaerobic threshold is another major factor allowing a faster pace or a longer run.

Oxygen cost of running

Since most distance runners and joggers rarely run at a pace commensurate with their VO_2max, the submaximal oxygen cost and efficiency of running are of prime importance. The submaximal oxygen cost of running is that volume (amount) of oxygen necessary to maintain a given speed aerobically. It is most often expressed relative to one's body weight (in millilitres per kilogram of body weight) so individuals of different sizes may be compared. Efficiency, or economy, of running is the oxygen requirement of a runner in comparison to other runners at the same speed. The runner using the least amount of oxygen at a given speed may be considered the most efficient.

Much research confirms the fact that the oxygen cost of running is directly related to the speed of locomotion. Our investigations appear to confirm the following equation for general use:

$$VO_2 \text{ (in)ml/kg/m} = 0.1999 \times \text{Speed (m/min)} - 1.9.$$

For example, if you run at 200 metres per minute (5 : 00 per kilometre), you require about 38.1 millilitres of oxygen per kilogram of your body weight every minute to maintain the energy production to keep you going at that speed.

Fractional utilisation coefficient

While the oxygen cost of running may index the relative efficiency of one runner to another, it does little to assess the stress placed on the body by the pace of the run. For this purpose the relative requirement of the individual's VO_2max is employed. This indicates the percent of VO_2max ($\%VO_2$max) at which the individual is exercising to travel at a given speed. For example, if our runner, who is travelling at 200 metres/minute and utilising 38.1 ml/kg/min of oxygen, has a VO_2max of 54.4 ml/kg/min, that pace is requiring about 70 per cent of the maximum aerobic capacity. This 70 per cent figure represents the level at which many authorities feel you must exercise in order for a training effect to result.

So important seems to be the $\%VO_2$ max at which the runner performs during a given steady state run that it may eventually surpass maximal aerobic capacity as a predictor of endurance performance. Not only does $\%VO_2max$ indicate the relative economy of running at a given speed, but it also indicates the potential of the individual to extend the effort to a maximum level. Since the relationship between running speed and oxygen requirement is linear, the fractional utilisation coefficient ($\%VO_2max$) indicates the degree to which a runner can increase the pace during aerobic running while maintaining the oxygen supply equal to the demand.

As a result of training, one's VO_2max is likely to improve 20–30 per cent while the oxygen cost of running may decrease by 5–7 percent, reflecting an improved efficiency. The $\%VO_2max$ at a given speed, therefore, will be reduced. Stated another way, you are able to run at a given pace with less stress or you may run at a faster pace to reach the same $\%VO_2max$ as before training.

Body composition changes

Among some of the most potentially profound changes resulting from endurance exercise are those occurring to the body composition. For our discussion, body composition refers to the amount and type of tissue making up the body. The most widely accepted model is the two-component scale which divides the body weight into a lean body mass (LBM) and a fat mass (FM). The LBM, although containing the skeleton, organs and other active tissues, is approximately 40–50 per cent muscle, and is used to represent the active, energy-producing tissues. The FM, on the other hand, is the inactive, storage tissue, that, while capable of providing a long-term energy pool, is best considered as excess baggage for runners. The ratio of the FM to the body weight is the percent fat ($\%fat$). Almost every runner has, at one time or another, been concerned with his or her body weight and its composition. While the major concern of the runner may be the body weight, more emphasis should be placed on its ratio of FM to body weight, i.e., $\%fat$.

The average untrained male and female have values of 13–15 and 23–25 per cent fat, respectively. International calibre male runners have relative fat values as low as 5–6 per cent, while their female counterparts may be around 8–10 per cent. Average male and female runners usually have values of 8–10 and 15–18 per cent respectively.

Numerous studies have shown that absolute (FM) and relative (%fat) body fat contents are inversely related to endurance running. That is, the more fat you have, the slower you run. Fortunately, the FM is a labile component that can undergo substantial change as a result of prolonged exercise. Because of the relatively high caloric demand of endurance running, the individual who engages on a regular basis is likely to reduce his or her FM, thus lowering the %fat.

Caloric cost of running

The caloric demand of running is directly related to body weight and independent of running speed. As the body weight increases, so does the energy demand to transport that weight during running. Although a runner travels faster and faster during training, it requires the same number of calories to cover a given distance. An accurate estimate of the energy cost of running may be derived from the equation:

$$\text{calories/mile} = 1 \cdot 25 \times \text{body weight (kg)} + 18 \cdot 7.$$

This is equivalent to approximately 0·95 calories per kilogram of body weight for every kilometre travelled. Therefore, given 7700 calories in a kilogram of fat, a 70 kilogram man would have to run 116 kilometres to lose that stored fat. Naturally, this is not accomplished in one day, but might easily be achieved in one week, provided the diet remains constant. Since medical and nutritional authorities recommend losing no more than a kilogram a week, exercise appears to be a safe and sound method of lowering the body weight, especially the unwanted fat content.

In order to lose weight with exercise, however, the supposition is made that one will maintain the dietary intake at the pre-exercise level. Several studies have shown that daily endurance running does not increase the appetite. Therefore, one must be careful not to rationalise that several miles of exercise should be rewarded by extra rations of cake, pudding or chocolates! After you reach the desired level of body fat, however, the exercise may allow you the luxury of extra calories without the penalty of extra fat accumulation.

Some people who run regularly and do not eat excessively may notice no significant decline in body weight. Changes are actually taking place, but they may be counteracting one another. The increased energy demand of running may be met by using up stored fat, thus lowering the FM. However, the muscles, in response to exercise, may grow slightly causing an increase in LBM. Therefore, weighing scales are not the best instruments for detecting the body composition changes resulting from your exercise programme. If your diet remains constant and your running remains regular, you will soon see the signs of reduced fat storage as you no longer pinch up excess fat at the waist line, on the hips and over the thighs.

Muscle fibre changes

Much attention has been focused on research literature identifying the types of muscle fibres a runner may have. Two general categories of muscle fibres have been identified, both of which may exist in the same muscle but in different proportions. One is the slow twitch (ST) fibre, often called a 'red' or oxidative fibre. It is red because of the staining procedure used in microscopic observation techniques. The stain is attracted to the enzymes of the aerobic mechanism and colours fibres with high oxidative capacities a dark red.

The other fibre is a fast twitch (FT) fibre, also known as a 'white' or glycolytic fibre. With a lower content of aerobic enzymes, this fibre does not attract the stain and hence appears colourless under the microscope.

It is rather clear that individuals with a greater number of ST fibres in their legs have greater VO_2max values and generally run better in the long distances. Unfortunately training appears to have little effect on changing FT to ST fibres. The percentage of ST and FT fibres in a runner's muscles is largely genetically determined and unalterable regardless of training method employed. It has been found, however, that FT fibres can increase their oxidative or aerobic capacity slightly with endurance training, thus moving towards the ST fibres at least in function. This may aid the distance runner in the final stages of a hard run or race. The significance of the changes is, as yet, uninvestigated.

While training will not alter muscle fibre type, it is well established that the aerobic enzymes in the ST fibres are increased in concentration with endurance work. The oxidative or aerobic capacity of the muscle is, therefore, increased, meaning that more work can be accomplished without producing lactic acid. In most individuals the improved VO_2max is due partly to increased cardiac output, i.e., pumping capacity of the heart, and partly to greater oxygen utilisation by the cells. As one ages, however, the changes resulting from training are largely confined to the cardiovascular system.

Summary

It is reasonable to assume that the physiological changes resulting from a running programme are multifactoral and interrelated. It is difficult to speak of changes in one area of the body without noting the changes in other areas. The universal consensus is that a carefully planned running programme individually tailored to a person's specific abilities and needs serves to improve almost all bodily functions.

More scientific information is coming forth each year to indicate that running may be preventive medicine. While no one is willing to state categorically that an exercise programme will prevent disease or prolong life, vigorous exercise individually suited to the person's needs may have wider implications for health than previously thought.

Each year science is producing thousands of new discoveries. The world of sports medicine and the effects of exercise on the body are so new that the full impact has not been felt. From available information, it appears that the exercising individual can lead a happier, healthier, more vigorous life than his sedentary counterparts.

3

Principles of Training

Activity is a biological necessity.

Hans Selye

The fitness runner should copy the training done by competitive athletes, lessening the quantity, lowering the speed and toning down the stress, to meet his/her own need and capacity. Running training is pretty well understood now, by experience and from the teachings of physiologists, and in practice the kinds of running that can be carried out shape themselves into six effective routines. All of these can be used by the fitness runner and, indeed, variety will add interest as well as produce comprehensive fitness.

In the past, weird training theories and practices abounded. Sweating, purging, eating undercooked meat, drinking sherry, not drinking when thirsty, were favoured nineteenth-century habits. A man would be sent out to run for twenty or thirty minutes, then be put into a feather bed and blankets, so that he sweated heavily, and then rubbed down with a dry towel. Strange notions of 'impurities', and of sweating these out of the body, made training for racing a form of punishment. Such ideas were propagated, for example, by Captain Barclay Allardyce of the 23rd Fusiliers, at the beginning of the last century, and Allardyce managed to walk 1000 miles in 1000 hours for a bet, in June–July 1809. The distances covered in running training, right up to the middle of the twentieth century were quite small, but some of the ancillary activities demanded of the athlete by his trainer could have created little in the way of enjoyment or strength. Allardyce punished himself and his followers; strangely, not so much in the amount of exercise (though the early 'pedestrians' certainly raced hard and long) as in the habits which were reckoned to support the actual training. Modern training places emphasis upon the quantity, type and pattern of running, and it is from the athlete's experience of steady-paced running, mixed-pace running, sprinting and hill-work, that the fitness runner, whatever his age or present condition, can learn. The sessions fall, as I have suggested, into six shapes. These may be adapted to meet individual requirements and circumstances.

First, and fundamentally most effective, is sustained movement, whether this be walking, jogging or running. When movement is continuous, most of the functions of the body will be touched and improved. A fit athlete will regularly run for anything up to an hour at sustained pace, looking upon this as his back-up mileage, upon which his specialised work will be founded. The Olympic champion, Lasse Viren, pointed out that after a period of hard racing he would move into many miles of steady running, to build himself up again. It is common practice for an athlete to have a long phase in winter, when he does only this kind of running, so that he will later be able to absorb and develop harder, faster running. At its very slowest, this is the popular 'jogging' or 'aerobic' movement, where the rate of running is slow enough to allow a person to get enough oxygen into the system to sustain movement without distress. The fitness runner might wish to rest here. But there are other kinds of running which can be nibbled at, to take the non-competitive runner beyond mere jogging fitness.

The sustained movement of steady-pace running, or of jogging or walking for that matter, can be broken up. An athlete uses 'interval' and 'repetition' running on the track, with numerous permutations of fast–slow running; or he uses the so-called 'fartlek' session, which is done over the country and is unplanned speed-play, with fast bursts at various distances thrown in along the way; or he does specific sprint and hill training. Each of these is available to the fitness runner. Each will make running for fitness much more fun, because there can be so much variety and challenge. Each is infinitely adjustable to meet individual requirements.

The purpose of these mixed-pace sessions is, to put the body under different stresses and through different ranges of movement. Whilst the fitness runner will, in most cases, not want to go as far as specialised running, he/she could valuably investigate and try the mixtures. For example, and once the preliminary stage (outlined in the next chapter) has been mastered, the enjoyable 'fartlek' method can be employed, especially if countryside is within reach, or even a short circuit through parkland or Forestry Commission land. Near where I live, there is such an area of FC wood, and it has a convenient wide track of about $1\frac{1}{2}$ miles circuiting the enclosed area. This track rises and falls all the way and is ideal for mixed-pace running, with the bonus of pleasant surroundings. Whatever your state of fitness, such an area is eminently useable. Survey it first, jogging and walking; then pick the stretches where you could raise speed a little, or run uphill. Each person adapts to his/her requirements and abilities. The 'fartlek' trainer gets several stretches at speed, and covers whatever distance is manageable or wanted. The overall effect is not severe, because running and relaxing combine. This kind of running-training was accurately called 'getting tired without feeling tired'. Fartlek can also be constructed imaginatively for use over a very short course, perhaps a half-mile or so. I call this activity 'circuitrees', because you plot a pleasant route, taking in some hill and you run a circuit, fartlek-style, which is through woodland and short enough for anyone to manage and to choose how many laps are covered.

If the mixed-pace running is done under more controlled circumstances, say on a track or a known road circuit, then the running comes nearer to being what the athlete calls 'interval' or 'repetition' running. Again, this can be adapted. A set distance is run, and a set interval allowed for recovery. The distance is made to suit the runner, as is the recovery phase. In the case of the fitness runner, the faster section would be very short – say 100 metres – and the recovery walk or jog generous. By making such a faster section very short, a little more speed can be injected. (The necessary warning is that any running that can justifiably be called 'fast', should be brought in carefully, to avoid muscle strain, or similar damage.) There is everything to be said in favour of doing not more than a few strides at speed, in the early stages of fitness running. It is easy to build up gradually. It is not so easy to conquer injury, which would mean going right back to the walking stage. Make haste slowly!

This point is even more relevant to any attempt at genuine sprint or hill running, where strain upon muscles and ligaments is considerable. Such strain may only be imposed upon fibres that are ready to take it, and then only gradually – gradually, that is, in terms of speed, duration and lift. Work from slow to fast over a period of many weeks. When you have raised your pace to recognisably fast running and can hold it for, say 20–30 metres, and are able to repeat this several times after jogging and walking, then begin to extend, until you manage 60–100 metres, which is enough. So is it enough to do such a session about once a week or so. This adds tone and strength to the muscles. To do such running on the hills is, naturally, more demanding, and a session of hill running should be introduced only when a modicum of sprinting has been accomplished. The angle and pitch of lower leg and foot, and the resultant pressure on the achilles tendon and the small muscles of the foot, are such that great care is needed. Never run before you can walk, and never run up hills until you can run on the flat. When you can run uphill, you will be able to add considerably to your fitness; the lift of the knees, the range of movement of the whole body, working against gravity, all repay with added strength, not to mention the sense of accomplishment when the fitness runner eventually finds that the hill is no obstacle. Hill-running is something which no competitive runner would omit from his plans.

Additionally, most athletes will regularly (at weekends, for example) break out and do a really long session, perhaps of two–three hours. There is a lesson here, too. The mental and physical results of this kind of freedom running are considerable. The fitness runner may not, in fact, be running for the bulk of such a session. Walking, plus jogging, plus relaxed running, plus the occasional mad burst, will be enough to create effects. It is the very thorough flushing that the body gets, the raising of heart-rate without strain, the continuous stretching of muscles, the taking in of oxygen; these functions are exercised, with just a bit of daring if the exerciser is normally limited to a routine life of work and travel and familiar territory. It is easy enough to carry a map, or just search out a different way each time. The whole operation is extremely enjoyable and there is every reason to try to form a group to do it. In those parts of the country where there are long-distance paths established, the activity is doubly enjoyable, since some of the best available ground is inevitably covered. To form and maintain a group of people who do this kind of trekking is to enhance other people's lives as well as your own.

One other kind of running can be recommended. This is the time-trial. A time-trial is no longer as much a part of running-training as it once was, but it is used and has much to recommend it. 'Joggers' very soon get used to running a particular stretch of ground and, therefore, like to see how long it takes to cover the distance. Finding out is a time-trial, which does not mean you have to put yourself under an obligation to the watch, but does mean that you create an additional incentive for extra effort and the resulting extra fitness. The time-trial can be employed on any course, for any distance. It is a very personal and independent measuring-stick, adding a great deal of interest to the activity.

Two extremely important principles underlie what has been said about types of training. First, any of the running, its quantity and quality, is adaptable by the individual, who is under obligation only to himself or herself; whether you walk, jog, stride or sprint, and whether you stay on your feet for ten minutes or ten hours, is entirely up to you, and will be based on what you find you can do. Second, and governing what has just been said, the principle of stress and recovery, of optimum load and, therefore, of sensible adaptation to that load, must suggest how much running can be done profitably. Present capacity is the guide. No sophisticated instruments are needed. You have the most sophisticated instrument of all, your body. Listen to it! This will allow proper judgement of the degree of severity of a session, in terms of time, distance and speed.

'Stress' is not only the stress produced by the act of taking exercise, just as 'recovery' refers not only to the period when no exercise is being taken. Stress that is physical is created by the sum total of one day's activity, slight though that may be for many people. Stress is also emotional, brought about by work for example; or social ('circumstantial' might be a better word), deriving from the whole, and recurring, routine of daily life – notably for those people who travel long distances to work. These are the stresses which limit the amount of direct physical stress, absorbed from running, which an individual can sensibly sustain. To take, again, the example of the competitive athlete, he must be free from too much general, unmanageable stress if he is to carry out his specialised training stress. It is impossible to commute long distances to work and be a highly successful athlete. So is it difficult to commute such distances and be a highly successful fitness runner, because the extra stresses will lessen the capacity for indulging the particular and healthy (because physical only) stress of running. The special point about the stress that comes from running is that it neatly counteracts the other kinds of stress, because being predominantly physical, it is actually relaxing in its final effect. To run is to get rid of some of the mental/emotional stresses picked up during the rest of the day. There is no magic or complete cure here, but a substantial palliative.

So, the fitness runner may vary and grade his running, and lodge it amongst his other activities. He need not be just a 'jogger'. Rather, he can be his own man in running, without any of the limits that jogging implies. However small his portion of running hard, up hills or on tracks, down the road or right across the country, he is free to develop whatever limit time and inclination propose. By extending his range of bodily movement beyond the locks and chains of jogging, he will be able to extend his fitness as far as is desired.

The primary training outlined above can get a useful boost from support training. This support training may have to replace the main exercise on occasions when shortage of time governs the day. Running-on-the-spot is effectively hard exercise, during which knee-lift can be varied. Sprinting-on-the-spot ('pattering'), with very little lift but a lot of speed, may be done by the fitness runner who has enough background to be sure of his muscle, tendon, ligament strength. You can also, with feet apart, lean forward and do 'arm running', which is a vigorous movement of the arms forward and backward. These exercises will give specific movement to limited groups of muscles and will slightly raise heart and breathing rate, with accompanying increased blood circulation. Three more static exercises, which are nevertheless useful muscularly, are slow knee-bending and straightening with back straight; leaning slowly back whilst sitting with the feet tucked under, say, a chair or bed; and adjustable press-ups, which may be done either leaning against a wall at arms' length, or on the back of a chair or desk, again at arms' length; or on the ground, in the classic 'press-up' position, depending upon your present strength. None of this compares with the abandon and total movement of closing the front door behind you and getting along the road or over the country at your own running pace. The exercises are better than nothing, not better than running. Most treatises on exercise over-rate them considerably, probably because they are convenient, easy and quick. What is too convenient, easy and quick is likely to give little in return. A half-hour's run is convenient and easy enough eventually. For fitness-effect it is unrivalled.

It is wise to remember, though, that such a valuable effect will not result from a couple of efforts. The assembly of a large number of runs over a period of time is what matters. Regulated, varied and built for a few weeks, these will break up the old unfitness. Maintained for months, and then indefinitely, the running-sessions will allow you to create and hold a kind and degree of fitness that you will not happily relinquish. The watchwords are: conscience and system. Given these, the body will adapt and progress. At any age, it will shed its old bad ways. When Bruce Tulloh ran from Los Angeles to New York (2876 miles in sixty-five days) in 1969, he commented on 'my faith in the adaptability of the body'. After forty days, and some 1700 miles, having endured quite a bit of muscular injury and discomfort, he found that his body worked perfectly, was fully adjusted. There is a lesson here, even if you only run four or five miles.

Conscience governs the successful athlete's training, and will, or would, govern the successful fitness runner's. The law of conscience is the best law anyway. It comes from inside the individual, it is only for him, and its rightness is almost guaranteed. It is not an easy law to obey, but it is a fruitful one. It comes from signing a treaty with yourself. The terms of the treaty, in this case, are completely selfish, but do nobody else any harm. They impinge upon your self-esteem and have, therefore, considerable force. They prompt and vitalise system; keeping plans deliberate and a clear horizon visible.

'System' covers what to do (dealt with in Chapter 4) and when and where to do it (Chapter 5). All that is written in those chapters is built upon the discussion in this one. Your system should employ the kinds of running exercise explained above and adapt them to your circumstance. Your conscience should ensure that enough is done, on your own behalf. Better still, the natural, inevitable pleasure of movement and fitness will turn running into something which your body wants and you want, so that there will be no effort involved; as the Olympic silver medallist, Lillian Board, remarked,

'To me, training every night is a foregone conclusion. It is a natural thing, just as natural as getting up in the morning or going to sleep at night.'

In competitive running, women are, physiologically, at a disadvantage when compared with men. Women have a smaller heart, less muscle, less haemoglobin, more fat. But in fitness running any comparison of women with men becomes completely irrelevant, because the runner is running for herself, not against anyone, and the fitness is her fitness, on her own terms. 'Bigger, stronger, faster' no longer has to mean anything, no longer matters; the man who runs for fitness is not compared with Ovett, Coe and Cram, so the woman need not be compared with any man. If she were, on any known criteria of fitness, she would probably be found most often to be superior. When it is a matter of condition rather than measurable performance, there is at the very least equality between the sexes.

Therefore, all kinds of running can be done by women fitness runners, at all kinds of personal levels, the stress and recovery belonging to each runner, rather than to some general rule or abstraction. A woman should find what is best for her.

There is, then, enormous scope for the fitness runner to vary and extend what he/she does. At each stage of progress, the right amount and type of running can be found and continual variety injected. Next, I would like to examine the practical situation more closely, indentifying what to do. This involves looking at how much running can be done, how to ease into the right quantity, and how to run.

4

What To Do

I go, and it is done.

(Shakespeare)

A healthy but untrained man or woman can walk as much as twenty miles, with no worse result than stiffness and blisters. That same person would find running, or even jogging, two miles extremely difficult, most probably beyond the immediate capacity. The long walk will require around six to eight hours, and is certainly recommended; the jog, and later the run, will take no more than twenty minutes once the early stages of running for fitness have been passed. It may be deduced that the stress of a twenty minute run, whilst different from that of the six hour walk, is more considerable and effective than the walk, as well as being more quickly obtained. In some ways, of course, the walk is superior; six hours in the fresh air are better than twenty minutes, whilst enjoyment of place and circumstance is likely to be enhanced by very slow, relaxed movement. But, purely in terms of applied stress to muscles, heart, circulation, in pursuit of eventual fitness, running must claim first place.

Knowing that you could walk, how far and how fast should you, at first, run?

These questions resolve themselves into: For how long? It is not necessary to measure miles or kilometres, yards or metres. Minutes are more obvious and even they should be taken as a guide and a measuring-rod, rather than as taskmaster or whip. Let us 'begin at the beginning'.

All but the very ill could walk for five minutes, or jog a few paces. Clearly, this would be next to useless as productive exercise. Wanting to make the body endure slight stress, so that recovery may create fitness, something between twenty and thirty minutes walking is necessary. The beginner is a convalescent in terms of fitness and he must stretch before getting up. When twenty–thirty minutes walking has been established as routine, and the process is easy, short stretches of jogging should be inserted. Listen in to your muscles, joints, nerves and organs. Do not impose upon them at this stage. Keep to the twenty–thirty minutes, because it is a manageable, undemanding length of time from every point of view, *and it will eventually be the period in which you can bracket enough running to bring fitness*. The first jogging phases need only last a few seconds, repeated as and when tolerable. Underplay, rather than overplay. You will, probably, be jogging for not more than a couple of minutes altogether in these early stages, and that will be enough to allow your body to begin to accept the gentle strain. You have, though, started in the direction of genuine fitness.

The principle is aiming to manage a half-hour of exercise, progressing from walking, to walking and brief jogging; later, to extending the jogs, later still to joining the jogging phases, and finally to raising the jog to a run. Chapter 6 deals, in practical detail, with this process, but there are several points which are allied to the question of what to do, and it is best to understand these before setting out.

First, it cannot be emphasised too often that training, at every level, is an individual affair. Interpreted, this does not mean that everyone should go out and do whatever he, or she, happens to prefer, because there are physiological truths and golden rules of training. Some routines of exercise will give better results than others. What it does mean is that our starting points are at different levels, our capacities infinitely variable, and our rates of progress singular and unpredictable. It follows that the amount of tiredness incurred is an individual response, so the amount of stress to be applied can only truly be known to the individual applying it. The obvious guide and teacher is the nervous system, which sends out signals, which we call pain. Acknowledge these at all times. Often they will be slight, and identified only as discomfort or effort. Beyond this, they will register as distress, an area which the fitness runner does not want to enter. It is not much fun, anyway!

Next, and developing the 'distress signal' idea, it is wise to remember that the fatigue (primarily chemical, affecting and inhibiting nerves and muscles) may be local or general. By 'local' is meant that which, for example, might affect the arm of somebody who saws wood, or the legs of somebody who climbs a ladder. Chemical changes in the active muscles soon signal fatigue and although the fatigue effect spreads and makes you breathe harder, such fatigue is safely limited. In running, even in jogging, the fatigue is much more general, as most of the body is being used to some degree. Therefore, take note, because demands are being made on general musculature and upon the heart. Excess strain upon either is not wanted, though boundaries will extend as running progresses intelligently, so that what was once hard becomes easy. The rule has always been: train, don't strain. Moving away from unfitness to fitness, there can be no hurry.

Furthermore, in a sensibly gradual programme, the amount of fatigue incurred as a result of a training session should be noted carefully. (A simple fatigue code can be employed, where $F1 = $ slight, and $F5 = $ very heavy, with appropriate gradings between.) Then note the amount of continuing tiredness, which is to say the layer that might be left after a night's sleep. And finally the amount which persists and builds. The first stage is inevitable and deliberately provoked. The second is a warning to be heeded. The third should not be allowed to occur, but might come from a combination of causes, many of which will have nothing to do with running. If the running done is relatively light (that is, relative to your own present capacity and feelings), there can be no danger of untoward fatigue. There should be continual progress. The fatigue level, though subjectively known, is an index.

Age and background must also affect for how long a person

can run at any stage of the programme. These are further reasons for accepting the individuality of each fitness runner and of what he or she does.

The age range of the fitness runner can be from fifteen to seventy-five; below fifteen there is little need to nurse or make fitness, above seventy-five the attempt to run is probably less valuable than walking. At all ages, the mixture of physical condition and age will control how far and how fast a person goes. For example, a twenty-year-old who has not grossly neglected himself will soon reach jogging level, whereas a fifty-year-old with no background of exercise should wait several weeks before any substantial distance is done above walking pace. If, or when, some months of exercise have been accomplished, the ideal twenty–thirty minute session may become, in both examples, a jogging session, but the effort/ speed within that period will remain very different for the two people. This is as it should be. You accept your own condition and ability.

If, with the half-hour mastered, a fitness runner wants to check how far he is travelling, and measure distance against time spent, to get an answer to 'How fast?', then he should do so. I would only argue that it does not greatly matter. What matters is, that there is continuing effort for about a half-hour and that this is developed from walking, through walking and jogging, through walking and sustained jogging, to continuous jogging, and later to running.

The idea of passing from walk to jog to run, and its significance as an indicator of fitness (that is, as the progression becomes possible) can be shown by referring to two elements in the mechanics of body-movement. When we pass from walking to jogging, we break contact with the ground; this action, of lifting and pushing the body-weight, is far more arduous than walking, and a fact of common experience. Then, when the very slow jogging movement is pushed to become a running action, the strain placed upon muscles, tendons, ligaments and joints, and the chemical reactions in the contracting muscle and the resultant demands upon the whole metabolism, are almost of a different order, even without coming near to sprinting. But, it is the eventual aim of the fitness runner to do a little true running, because the range of movement is extended and the body's general strength and suppleness vastly improved. The convenient point about fitness running is, that you go just as far as you want. Many non-competitive runners/joggers may not wish to go to the stage of proper running, just as many pianists may not want to play difficult pieces, yet such an achievement is there to be had. The exhilaration of running, particularly of running short, fast stretches, is not to be missed, and merely lies a little further on!

Part of this process, and a means of achieving the physical freedom which is presented by running, is learning *how* to run. Running may have been a natural act once, but it is not so any longer. The beginner in fitness running is likely to be especially clumsy and lumbering, and needing to observe three cardinal principles of good running – relaxation, rhythm and fluency. Self-taught, by practice and imagination, running which is relaxed, rhythmic and fluent becomes not only effective mechanically, but very pleasurable. Even amongst athletes, skilled running is rare.

Relaxation begins during walking. A conscious choice is made to let the tension fall out of muscles and it is not so difficult to walk loosely, in a slovenly manner which yet does not allow limbs to go all over the place. Moving into a jog, the relaxation is kept and the control of the direction of arms and legs is still deliberate; for example, feet and knees go straight forward, arms and hands move quite close to the body and fairly high. There is nothing fussy, artificial or strained about this. If, or when, the running movement is attained, so must this easy control be. Now rhythm and fluency dominate. The secret lies in noticing the complete cycle of movement involved. It is felt as a wheel moving. There are no jerks, no breaks in the cycle. The action flows and the sound of feet is rhythmic. Interestingly, a runner usually finds that he has a tune in his head, put there by the rhythm and difficult to dislodge. Keep it, because it helps.

Such running is not fatiguing, for the minimum of tension and the maximum of fluency allow a proud speed without pressure.

This is also the place at which to mention several quick, supplementary activities which will boost and aid what the running promotes. Although runners like to run primarily, and running is comprehensive enough to give the desired fitness, circumstances do often inhibit activity, or may on occasion offer special chances of, for example, gymnasium 'circuit training'. These are opportunities not to be missed, though the same caution should be observed as with the opening shots of the running campaign. You cannot go into a gym, jump about on benches, climb ropes, hang from wall-bars, etc., and expect to avoid pulled muscles. When running is impossible (which should be rarely), better than nothing would be digging the garden, or sawing wood, or posting your letters at a distant box one at a time, even shopping at speed. Somehow, get the twenty or thirty minutes of movement. Usually, the fitness runner will find a way of getting his run. The nineteenth-century athlete, W. G. George, even invented what he called his '100 Up' exercise, which was done indoors when too much work took his time. A hundred running strides on the spot can be quite effective when the knees are raised, and they may be varied in speed, quantity and range very simply.

Therefore, a profitable half-hour is the aim. It may take months to reach a half-hour of actual running, but that is the target and, to an extent, the motive. Slow progress is sure progress and there is no reason to consider failure. Once the half-hour is attained, it will be a very important part of your life, not happily relinquished and giving a large measure of fitness. The pace, stress and range of movement all grow with and from the individual and are met by him only, not measured by some absolute criterion and not imposed from outside. Eventually, fluent and enjoyable running will be possible. The next questions are where and when?

5

How Often—Where and When?

The night is dark and I am far from home.

(Cardinal Newman)

There is truth for the fitness runner in the words of one Olympic champion: 'I made a commitment to myself and I was not going to let anything stand in the way.' Finding the time and place to run, and finding them often enough to produce results and satisfy intentions is the central practical problem for any athlete, the test of his own commitment and the proof of his motivation.

To develop fitness is to follow a long road. But you cannot read a book in five minutes, or master more than one bar of music; anyway, the process is enjoyable, so the length of time it takes is a bonus rather than a penalty. If you know what kind of running you want to do, the next step is to work out how often, where and when to run. 'How often?' is the step on which most people fall down, and 'Where?' and 'When?' provide the excuses.

A decent level of fitness could eventually be achieved by running every other day. The pattern and rhythm of alternate days of exercise and recovery is very effective. Clearly, this pattern depends upon how much is done in a session, and how hard that running is. A quick, light session has little effect and therefore, done every other day, would allow scant progress. The pattern of stress and recovery does demand a level of stress that can be felt. If the beginner is walking and jogging for a half-hour, the alternate-day rhythm is going to be valuable. It is the minimum, though. To lose only every third day would be better still. The clue to attitude lies here, and proposes that every day is a running day; then the occasional missed day is not significant.

The most practical approach is to sit down for a few minutes on Sunday, look at the coming week and judge which days will allow serious running. Very few will not. So, the question becomes, 'How often this week?', and the answer is 'at least five times'. If the answer were 'every other day', you could be satisfied that such a routine would help. What the true runner always feels, though, is that he will make time for the thing he enjoys and which rewards him. To run every other day is to deny yourself the pleasure of running every other day! And, as more running is done, so the desire and capacity increase. How often you run begins to determine how often you run. Once the hill has been climbed, the mountain looks inviting.

Normally, Saturday and Sunday allow considerable freedom so that if Friday is taken as an entry to that freedom – for example, in the knowledge that the Friday evening run can be followed by a relaxed start to Saturday – nearly half the week is easily made available. How often you exercise during a week is a question of how often do you exercise between Monday and Thursday.

'Where?' and 'When?' must be linked. Where I am at a particular time governs when I can run. It also governs the practical details, such as whether a shower is on tap, and whether I shall have to sit in a warm room immediately afterwards. Again, it is usually possible to punch a hole in the day somehow. At the end of the last century, a London journalist, J. E. Fowler-Dixon, got himself quite a few headlines by his running-training and racing. Stuck in London, Fowler-Dixon nevertheless trained for the very long road races, and managed records up to 100 miles in both running and walking. His training regularly involved him in hiring a 'cab' (horse-drawn taxi) in Regent's Park, changing and depositing his clothes in the vehicle, and using it as a pacemaker. He lived to the age of ninety-three, and had run a mile in 7 mins 07 secs on his seventy-first birthday. Modern workers in cities such as London manage also to find room and time to run; indeed, I counted more than thirty one afternoon in Vancouver, whilst the Mount Royal Park in Montreal boasts a sign which bans traffic and allows runners. There is a time and a place to be found, if the searcher intends to find them. I have run in Islington High Street and on the coast of Newport, Oregon, and although it would be easy to state a preference there, the point is that if you want to run, you will find the time and the place.

'Where?' also covers the question of variety. To run always on the same stretch of road is to court boredom. Even to run always on the same stretch of beautiful countryside is perhaps to make the process too much of a routine. Variety induces pleasure, which is persuasive. Therefore, try to pick a different place often. Even follow a route in a different direction, or chop it into smaller sections. Best of all, search out new routes and store up the favourite ones for really free running at the weekends, when the 'fartlek' can be employed, or the very long 'trek'. Sometimes, the course can be a hilly one, sometimes one which allows some faster bursts. I find, still, that running repeated 100 metre stretches on a track is exhilarating as well as strengthening, and the occasional visit to a track helps to add variety. It is also well worthwhile to drive a few miles occasionally, to find the best, or just different, territory.

Where you run reminds you of the need for some care with surface and with shoes. Too much road, for example, is not good; whilst the well-heeled shoes needed on road may prove useless on the muddy tracks of a wood. These are points which require a moment's thought the night before. If, as H. G. Wells noted, 'Forethought is an expensive commodity', injury can prove even more expensive, and the frustration of not being able to run properly because of wrong shoes in the chosen place, is enough to spoil the pleasure and weaken results.

Probably, place is as important as anything in the growth of pleasure in running and, therefore, in the wish to continue and develop. For example, I know that within about an hour of writing this sentence, I shall be running through Mereworth

Woods, near Tonbridge, Kent. These are mixed, deciduous woods, with a lot of chestnut, and they are large enough to allow a seven-mile lap, which in turn allows many variations of direction and distance. The paths are wide, if muddy, and the place mostly deserted. The air is fresh and the sense of freedom welcome. So, to run there is total pleasure. The same could not be said about every place, especially since mankind seems intent on spoiling most of the woodland; but it will be possible, even in a city, to find somewhere which, in itself, accommodates and provokes the pleasure and satisfaction of running. Similarly, the context of a track, which is not likely to be scenically or aesthetically persuasive, has an atmosphere and a sense of purpose which create particular satisfaction for the runner. The measured circuit of the track can be as much fun as the haphazard route through the trees. A fitness runner should look for woods, tracks, roads, beaches, or any other places where running can be enjoyed.

Incidentally, there is no need to hide! There seems to be, in the newcomer at least, a sense of embarrassment, almost shame, about going out and running on the road, or indeed where anyone may see you. It is a sad comment on our way of living, that the runner should still be looked upon as eccentric, rather than as the person in whom a kind of sanity is vested. Everything from mild amusement through to mockery and even outright contempt is displayed by the public in so many countries (though this is happily now changing). One of the responsibilities of the runner is to show the flag to the smirking public and to have more of them join you, since they cannot beat you. The tubby beginner might be justified in slipping out under the net of darkness for his first few runs, but surely he is to be congratulated, not derided? Knowing this, he should have the extra bit of courage to flaunt his efforts, and perhaps convert his unconvincing critics. Straight down the High Street is not very practicable, but it would not be a bad move. Done daily, such action might breed familiarity rather than contempt. It has been the unusual nature of the activity in modern societies which provoked the flimsy derision, and the public highway is the place to knock that derision, which is probably shallow anyway. If in doubt, get others to run with you. Eventually, there will be more of us than of them.

For most people, there will be three times a day when running can be done, and there will be freedom to choose at the weekend. Since we must run either early in the morning, at mid-day or in the evening, the best scheme is one which creates variety. For example, knowing that Saturday and Sunday are fairly free, a session can be arranged on Friday evening; therefore, Thursday could be left out or kept for a short lunch-time run or walk; and Monday, Tuesday and Wednesday used very deliberately with, say, an early morning run on Monday, a lunch-time one on Tuesday, and an evening on Wednesday. Experience shows that this method of changing the time of day used for your run is most acceptable, because you do not then always block off a particular part of every day from other uses. Of course, some people like the persuasion of routine and will want to run at the same time every day. It remains an individual matter. I find that the freedom of change is important.

You may learn that, like very many runners, you cannot happily exercise in the early morning soon after getting up. Pulse-rate is then low, muscles have had little movement for several hours, the brain is dulled or dreamy, the eyes heavy. All argues against running. Some people break out of this state very quickly, but most of us find action immediately on rising irksome. Since punishment is not the purpose of fitness running, and since (especially in winter) there is little fun in dragging a reluctant body out, it may be that the early morning is written off. There is a case, though, for trying once a week at that time of day. It frees the rest of the day and it gives you an ounce of self-control, which is not a bad thing when you are trying to get fit. Even for those of us who are not made for early morning exercise, the rising sun in spring and summer is an encouragement as well as an experience. If you are lucky enough to have bathing facilities at work, and not to have to catch a train, then the system is simple. Dress in running gear, stow clothes in a bag, eat little or nothing, drive to the nearest wood or park on the way to work, have a half-hour run, go on to work, shower, change, have a flask of drink and a marmalade 'butty' – and make a good start to the day.

When mid-day is used, possibilities must again be infinite, and particular to the individual. Even in a city, by taking sandwiches a mid-day half-hour can be found for running. It must be a rule not to run too soon after eating, and it is never very enjoyable to eat fully too soon after running, so the ideal arrangement is to go for a run, wash and relax for a while, and then eat lightly. Others may eventually join you, and your need for a fraction more time may be tolerated. At worst, sandwiches can be eaten on returning to work. In practice, most jobs allow some kind of manipulation and freedom, even if only once a week.

Running in the evening is easiest (and in summer more comfortable), though your own domestic routine may complicate matters, or the travelling you need to do, or the winter darkness. Again, there is value in not trying to run at the same time every day, and thereby easing arrangements with the rest of the household. Always to delay an evening meal, or always to come home and go straight out again, is not the way to popularise running for fitness. As has been suggested, it might be convenient to have one evening run and this might be with a group or club, to give your morale a boost. The permutations are many, of time and place. For example, arrangements with friends or fellow-travellers may make it possible to get a lift within three or four miles of home, so that the distance can be run, and clothes dropped at your house by the chauffeur. This sort of arrangement is not difficult.

Because 'When?' depends on 'Where?', it will be the lucky few who live at exactly the convenient distance from work, travel by the most practicable route and vehicle, or have the most helpful friends. These lucky few will be able to do what many athletes do, which is to run to and/or from work, evolving numerous routes and distances, saving a lot of petrol money or bus fares, and injecting a period of freedom into the day. Once you have worked out where certain clothes (and keys) have to be at given moments, and got over the early mistakes which are bound to be made, this routine of using your own legs to travel, is unrivalled. Combined with the trick of having a folding bike to go in the boot of your car and be left at whichever end of the journey you want it, this type of travelling opens all sorts of possibilities and must create a high level of fitness. The whole programme is worth serious consideration and plotting. In the very early days, a combination of walking, running and cycling is favourite; gradually, as fitness emerges, a sustained run will be possible once or twice a week.

Out of these possible schemes, according to the needs of the individual but with resolution and imagination, a weekly plan can be forged. You will, quite easily, be able to work out when and where to run, maintaining variety, seeking new times and places, experimenting with your own special arrangements.

With Saturday and Sunday comes freedom to run where and when you like. Enjoyment still comes from variety of time and place. Remember, too, that the weekend offers a chance of increasing both the quantity and quality of running, and therefore of increasing fitness. Experiment with sustained running, with hills, and with 'fartlek'. One of the results will be to increase the ambition and pleasure attached to the following week's running, giving the whole continuing process more momentum.

How often, where and when you run depends ultimately on motivation, on wanting to run and to reap the benefits. This must be especially true of 'How often?'. There is no sudden, slick method of persuading yourself. If the first impetus came from an awareness of your lack of fitness, continuing demands imagination and will be encouraged by experience (which is why choice of place is so important). The process is cumulative; only get started and the most difficult phase will be over. This is, anyway, the right time to start, because more and more people are discovering running for fitness and there is bound to be somebody or some group that can be contacted, for encouragement. Yet, whatever incubation takes place, the desire to run and be fit lodges in a secret place within the individual. No formula or advice is going to reach down into the 'throng and stack of being'; no neat verbal maxim is going to get a response or maintain the process. This only comes from getting your feet on the road or in the grass, through the trees or round the track. And in those places will be found the encouragement.

6

Getting Started

And we,
Light half-believers in our casual creeds,
Who hesitate and falter life away,
And lose tomorrow the ground won today.

(Matthew Arnold, *The Scholar Gipsy*)

If you are over the age of thirty, and particularly if you have no background of regular exercise and are over-weight, do not contemplate running until you have been checked by a doctor. This is an unbreakable rule for the beginner. And it does mean making an appointment with the doctor, rather than slipping in at the end of the queue at a busy surgery. Explain to the doctor what you intend to do, so that he will check your heart, because that is the vital muscle! If he clears you, you need not see him again for fifty years.

Age must be a crucial factor governing the way that a fitness runner starts training. At thirty, there should be a fair amount of suppleness and quick potential; at forty, the early stages of exercise will require stubborness; at fifty and beyond, preliminary efforts must be protracted and very gently graded. There are plenty of people who have taken up running after the age of seventy, so there really is no barrier other than illness or structural damage.

First, buy a pair of running shoes. Plimsoles, or 'sneakers', will not do. They will merely allow foot, leg or back damage. Most muscle, tendon, ligament injuries will start because of carelessness at foot/ground level. Therefore, get shoes which are built for running. The cheapest, even though they may be called 'training' shoes, also will not do, because they will lack quality protective heel and sole layers and will have sub-standard uppers, probably too stiff. Your primary investment, which is in shoes, may seem expensive, but is not. A good pair will last and be comfortable (see Chapter 10).

Second, and at the same time, begin to lose weight and to do some indoor exercise. A combination of exercise and very slight reduction in food will allow gradual loss of excess fat. There is no case for fasting, or for dramatic sacrifice. Food is fuel. Short-term fasting will reduce strength, just at the time when a little stress is being applied to the body. It may take a mile of steady running (which lies some months ahead) to use about a hundred calories, so that regular exercise and a slight reduction in the more obvious and unnecessary food, such as the over-full spoon of sugar, the second piece of cake, or the third potato, will allow a small, steady loss of fat.

What matters always is the balance between food intake and exercise; increase exercise and decrease food, with the delightful prospect of being able eventually to enjoy the second bit of cake and the third potato, when exercise has become regular and hard enough to wipe out their effects. Also, do not be fussy about food. We know when we have eaten enough, or when we have eaten too much starch. In general, eat comprehensively and without fads.

By 'indoor training', I mean some preliminary stretching and jogging, and a little localised strengthening. If muscles have not been seriously used for some time, it will be wise to do some toe-touching, first when sitting and later when standing; some knee-raising, arm-stretching and swinging; and some stomach and shoulder exercise. The stomach exercise is simply done by placing the feet under a bed or armchair and leaning back, to an angle which demands a bit of effort, holding that position and sitting up again, or by lying flat on your back and raising the heels off the ground, with legs straight. Shoulders can be exercised by standing with the feet apart, leaning slightly forward, and 'running' with the arms. This also helps the stomach and the chest. A small amount of on-the-spot jogging is valuable, before you venture onto the road or country. This jogging will allow you to sense the strength of the feet, heels and lower legs particularly, and to control the amount of stress being put on the legs. It will also allow some of the inevitable early soreness to be provoked and shifted before the proper walking/running sessions begin. And wear running shoes, so that they settle on the feet.

This preliminary indoor exercise is something of an image of what should precede any later running session. The fittest athlete is not going to charge straight into his running; rather he is going to walk, amble, jog, stride, jog . . . . and so on, to give his body a chance to accustom itself to the demands made on it. The unfit apprentice runner must be even more guarded in his approach. The heart-rate responds to the action of the musculature, and common sense (certainly common experience) tells us that coaxing is better than sudden assault.

More often stated than observed, is the maxim 'train, don't strain'. The fitness runner should observe it. At the very beginning, knowing that you can walk for a half-hour, do just this, but allow yourself to get the feel of relaxed running, in stretches of not more than twenty or thirty metres. If you have to work hard for these, or if you feel excessively tired and breathless afterwards, keep the number down; the number must be an individual affair, in any case. The absolute key is to find out what you can do by doing it. If you can only walk, then walk. After a few sessions of walking, the short easy runs will be possible, because the body will be fractionally stronger. This must happen! There is a reaction and a reward, which is the point of the activity.

A few targets should be set up right from the start. For example, aim eventually to be able to run easily eight times in the half-hour. If you can manage four times at first, there is the immediate target, which is five times, and the next, which is six. When the eight are mastered, you are running about 200 metres, which is good. Fitness is on the way. The next target is to lengthen the stretches. This will be a process which demands regularity and time. For the completely unfit beginner, to get from the first walking session to the ability to run easily eight times for about 100 metres, may take a couple of months. If it takes four, no matter; there are plenty available. One American, who started exercising seriously at the age of seventy, took six months to master a three-mile easy run. Later he became capable of twenty miles a week. There can be no hurry. To hurry, or force the body is to make a fundamental mistake and probably to deny yourself success, if only because there has to be ample recovery, which in turn implies the right amount of effort.

There will come a time when you can run for the full half-hour. That is the main target.

Muscle soreness is to be expected in the early days. Don't blame the exercise; blame the previous lack of it. Treat the symptoms of your former neglect respectfully, though. Adequate shoes must be worn always, or there will be a risk of actual muscle injury. Rest a day or two, if there is extreme soreness. I recall a sudden burst of enthusiasm which persuaded a barrack-room friend to run the perimeter of an airfield with me. He had done no running for years and a day later he was in the station sick-room, virtually unable to walk and, presumably, suffering from several hundred tiny muscle pulls. His attitude was sane enough, but his action not intelligent (I should have told him, but did not wish to spoil a good thing). Make haste slowly. Find exactly the right amount of walking/running for yourself, upon which to build week by week.

The mental picture to carry is of a long, slender line (which is the half-hour of movement); on this you emboss, at intervals, short thick lines (which are the running stretches). Week by week, the thick lines are lengthened, until the slender line becomes the shorter. Eventually, this slender line is completely covered by the thick lines, which now indicate a continuous, albeit slow run. When that stage is reached there is good cause for celebration, so go for a run.

This could be the stage you were seeking. But before resting content as a 'jogger', consider how much more fitness and satisfaction there could be. Look back to Chapter 3. Which of the kinds of running might now be done? The point is, if you are going to run easily for a half-hour, and have made the effort to do so, there is every reason to continue the experiment, particularly to ring the changes and keep the activity interesting and challenging.

For example, the easiest, the mixed-pace 'fartlek' run is a slight advance on the maintained 'jog', and can always be tailored by and for the individual. The practice is to raise pace over particular stretches of ground, including a hill or two. The effort on these stretches will be fractionally harder, because fractionally faster, longer or stronger, than the steady run. Or, the fitness runner who has graduated might try a deliberate session of his own level of sprinting, repeating stretches of about 100 metres at slightly beyond the usual pace, but remembering here, particularly, the importance of limbering up first. Simplest of all, is the attempt to cover more distance in the half-hour, or to cover the known distance in less than a half-hour, or to add five or ten minutes to the usual run. Before looking at ways of measuring progress, and thus of making progress, here is a skeleton programme for the beginner, summarising what has been argued so far and what may be practically manageable.

First Plan
(to allow acquisition of basic running fitness)

Number of days training:	every other – therefore fifteen per month
Time spent:	half an hour per session
Proportion of running to walking at start:	10 per cent running
Number/length of running stretches:	20–30 metres done eight times
Method of progress:	gradually extending length of the running stretches
Period of progress which may be expected:	two months to reach 50 per cent running; four months to reach easy running for half-hour; six months to have established this

7

Measuring Progress

I used to like examinations. I used to love the
test.

(Ron Clarke, holder of twenty-one
world track records)

The idea of progress does not presume that there is some
final target to be reached. The only standard that might be
currently set would be the world record for a particular
distance, and this is no concern of the fitness runner, unless he
is a spectator at the sport of 'track and field'. But, change which
pleases can be measured and the measurement is an incentive
as well as an indicator. If you are pleased by the change in your
physical fitness, you will probably want to check that change
occasionally. There is no need to go to elaborate lengths.

The possibility of progress may be presumed, so long as
illness or injury does not interrupt. Sports that do not demand
particular skills are sports in which progress is directly related
to effort. Running is such a sport. This is not to say that
progress will be dramatically fast. But there will be changes in
the physical condition, so long as a regular, designed physical
effort is being made.

These hoped-for changes are built upon graded running,
which is simply attained and inevitable as the weeks pass.
Walking and running progress to running and walking, then
to running, then to slightly faster running; there is no need to
prophesy, to state exactly what distance or pace will be attemp-

ted or attained. Rather, it is a case of the body *allowing* more
to be done, in terms of distance and speed, with a guarantee
that the allowance will grow with time.

What helps greatly is having a series of targets. These range
from the first one, which is to complete a half-hour's exercise
with eight short stretches of running, to achieving a new time
for a set course. The targets should be practical and they
should tell you something, rather than being just arbitrary.
An arbitrary target would be, for example, to run 365 miles in
one year, or 1986 miles in 1986, or 28 miles in a particular
February. This is a habit nearer to astrology than to intelligent
running, because 365 miles in a year, or 365 kilometres in a
year, or whatever, bears no necessary relationship to the work-
ings of your body. It is a convenient figure, plucked from a
calendar, and it will not make a useful target.

The idea of a target connects to the idea of progress, which
in turn connects to the special, daily physical condition of an
individual person. To plant an arbitrary mileage figure upon
an individual is to ignore the particular condition and stage of
development of that individual. What has to be done is, that
a known course which has been run before, should be run at
regular intervals, so that the time taken can be recorded. For .
example, once a month (an arbitrary interval!) the course
originally used for the half-hour attempt could be run and
walked, and eventually run, and this effort timed. Thus you
will find out what the University of Oregon coaches call your
'date pace'; that is, the pace you are capable of on, say, 1 June,
when you first time yourself. You could then have a 'goal pace',
which would be anything faster than the achieved 'date pace'
and which you might hope to establish on 1 August. The
target is yours, because the course is yours, the effort yours,
and the original measurement a measurement of your particular physical condition. You can go on from there, almost
indefinitely, certainly optimistically.

The 'fatigue index' can be used to indicate how much effort
a measured run cost you. It is not an objective, scientific
measurement, but it is no less valuable for that. Incidentally,
in the early stages of running/walking, when you are not really
used to hard exercise, you will probably exaggerate the suffer-

ing, as you beat the ends of nerves that have been dormant, with muscles that complain! Since it is very wise to play safe, this exaggeration will be to your benefit. The fiercer, more imaginative efforts and the tougher responses can be left until later. A significant practical pointer to effort and fatigue is pulse-rate, at rest and at various intervals after different efforts.

Resting pulse-rate should drop as exercise is established and improved. The heart becomes stronger and slower. This is a measure of success. The other interesting measures are those made directly after running and occasionally after that; for example, an hour afterwards, three hours afterwards, and the morning after, that is directly on waking. As a rough guide, pulse at 120 beats per minute indicates a considerable degree of effort. Therefore, if such a rate is reached with very little running done, fitness cannot be acceptable. Walking should raise the pulse only slightly, jogging noticeably and running sufficiently. Keep an exact note of the varying pulse-rates you have. After a time, the picture will emerge and some guidance will be established. The slower pulse will be observed, with a lower ceiling for comparable efforts and times. It is, of course, all somewhat academic. Measurement tells you what is happening; it does not make it happen.

Pulse, the direct recorder of heart work, must be the crucial physiological measurement. Degree and rate of recovery confirm what the pulse says. If heavy fatigue is experienced and if it lasts into the day following exercise, then the exercise was too hard. Tiredness will occur, but a night's sleep must remove this. Fatigue might build up over a few days and relaxation of the running effort (not stopping) will remove this. Exhaustion is the competitive athlete's privilege and should not be experienced by a fitness runner. You are in a very practical situation, where the body signals its condition and should be listened to, so that you have a clear idea of how much you have done and how much you can do.

These subjective reactions should be respected. In some ways, they are superior to any objective measurements. Anyone who has coached athletes honestly will admit that, even with a stop-watch or other technology, and with knowledge of an athlete's current ability and performance, assessment of degree of effort and, therefore, of degree of physiological stress, is not possible from outside, certainly not from outside a really sophisticated laboratory. The person inside the body knows best. This is why it is unwise to set a rigid schedule for an athlete. Similarly, progress will be made by a fitness runner who has an outline idea of each session but listens to his own body and to its signals of stress and recovery. The runner is the 'ghost in the machine'. Whilst he needs to be encouraged and helped, he cannot finally be told. Luckily, there are no absolute criteria for the measurement even of muscle capacity – only the example of what has been achieved, against which we may get some notion of our own level.

The practical measurement, then, is that which an individual can make in terms of course/distance/time; several courses/ distances/times; and on special courses such as the track or hills. All measurements so carried out will be measurements of individual progress. You have succeeded if amongst those you beat is the man, or woman, you were a month ago.

It is best to have at least four courses on which to assess your progress. The practical target is then the one which requires you to beat your previous time for the selected course. By having four courses, you can try a short one, taking about ten minutes and allowing a very firm, controlled effort; a longer one, taking about twenty minutes and requiring good sustained effort; one that takes about the half-hour, which is the one you started on and can now beat; and an accurately measured lap of a track, which you might be able to visit occasionally.

A simple diary, to log running done, degree of fatigue produced by each session, achievements and aims, can easily include a table (see below) for recording the course times. Merely state when and where the run was achieved, and the time it took on that particular day; a year or two later, this will be interesting reading. A particularly useful trick is to have, on the longest course, three or four distinguishable places at which the time can be noted. For example, I know on my Mereworth Woods course that, on 14 April 1978 I passed the gate by the timber yard in 17 minutes, the gate off the main track in 28 minutes, and reached the road in 38 minutes. This spread differed from the previous 14 April; it was slower overall and the last section took much longer as comparative unfitness made the final stretch difficult. Every year counts, too! Thirty years of regular running have not, though, removed the desire to check how long it takes me to run a particular course, or to believe that it will not take so long next year. I suppose it would be sensible to grow up, but I do not have the slightest inclination to stop recording distances and times. It is very likely that a fitness runner who is new to the activity will catch this particular disease. It is harmless enough.

This is the point at which to give some criteria by which the newcomer can judge his standard. I would again stress that it is your own progress, related to where you were when you started and where you were last month, etc., that matters most. The examples given in Chapter 9 are impressive and encouraging. Here, it is useful just to indicate how the stop-watch describes pace and how athletes measure accomplishment. For any sort of accuracy it is necessary to go to a track, where the 400 metres lap is always 400 metres, so that the time taken to run a lap is an undeniable measure.

Complex and extended tables, points systems, percentages, and so on are not included in this book. A combination of distance, time, 'date pace', feeling of difficulty or ease sensed, level of fatigue apprehended, rate of pulse, will be an ample guide to what is happening, especially when this combination is regularly noted.

Experience shows that a fitness runner who can complete the 400 metre lap in two minutes has achieved a useful degree of strength, both muscular and organic. Eight minutes for the four laps (which, on the metric track, is 9·35 metres over a mile) is, therefore, a substantial test in the early days. (It is, of course, not more than a 'warm-up' pace for the athlete.) Eventually to complete fifteen laps in your half-hour would be an accomplishment on which to build seriously, if you wish. Again, this sustained pace is not impressive to the true runner, whilst many men and women over the age of fifty, and a handful over the age of seventy, have completed the 26+ miles of a marathon at a faster average mile pace than eight minutes. However, it remains a reasonable and attainable aim and a fair measure of fitness. Most citizens could not do it. In 1978 the British Army was using eight minutes per mile pace as a yardstick by which to assess the physical fitness of the majority of its personnel.

What you accomplish, how far you eventually take your level of fitness, must depend upon your attitude. As Shakespeare's Henry V says: 'All things are ready if our minds be so.' Once you have experienced a high level of physical fitness, you will be reluctant to sacrifice it, because it enhances every day. So there is a natural momentum to the process. Activity increases the desire for activity. Accomplishment allows further accomplishment. Imagination creates an escape, which becomes reality on your various courses. Difficulties will arise, but can be met and moved.

Table of courses

Course A		Course B		Course C		Track	
Date	Time	Date	Time	Date	Time	Date	Lap Times

8

Overcoming Difficulties

'I'm very brave generally,' he went on in a
low voice, 'only today I happen to have a
headache.'

(Lewis Carroll,
Alice Through the Looking-Glass)

The Russian pianist, Vladimir Ashkenazy, said that everything
is difficult once you have decided to do it. The difficulties
which a fitness runner is likely to face are not weighty, though
there may be plenty of them. They gather, because the process
takes time. They can be roughly grouped, and discussed as
physical, mental, domestic and social. Once they are acknowledged, they can often be thwarted and their bad effects
avoided.

Physical difficulties will be injury, illness, lack of proper
sleep or food, and weather; these difficulties can be avoided,
accommodated, managed or ignored.

Almost always, injury sustained whilst running will be an
injury to the leg or foot. Serious injury caused by a fall or a
collision does not come within the bounds of this discussion,
because such injury is not solely related to running and would,
in any case, be a matter for professional medical opinion.
If you do not run, you are unlikely to suffer muscle pulls or
ligament strains (though the worst case of torn Achilles I ever
saw was sustained by a man who slipped off a door-step). The

painful Achilles tendon, the torn hamstring, and the niggling foot injury are nasty presents for the runner, but they are mostly avoidable because they are usually acquired carelessly. We come back to the motto: train, don't strain. Sudden demands made upon muscles that lack tone or strength will, logically, force damage. Protracted, though weaker, demands may have the same effect. Therefore, create and allow only the right amount of stress for your present condition. If anything, play safe and move forward gradually. If injury is suffered, go back to walking, be patient and prepare to build again slowly and deliberately. Nature will not be hurried. And make sure that your running shoes are in perfect condition, affording you the necessary protection. Trouble starts underneath the feet.

It would be a lucky runner who could get through a year without illness of some kind. But, running is a prescription for health, so any illness is likely to be of the common cold or 'flu variety. These should be treated with respect. Never run if your temperature, or pulse, is unusually high, because such an increase must be a warning that the body is struggling against an infiltrator. There is no sense in making that struggle more difficult by hard exercise. The consequences could be serious. Patience is the virtue in this circumstance and it may be a week before a run can be taken. If you know your regular pulse and have checked its pattern over a long period, it will be easy to judge when something is wrong and when recovery is complete, apart from the usual, obvious, symptoms. Your knowledge of pulse-rate and pattern will give early warning, anyway; an increase, say on waking, will always indicate either that you did too much the day before, or that a germ is being harboured. Read the signs. After illness, return to running gradually, testing reactions daily and judging the tolerable quantity of exercise by the amount of stress produced.

A fitness runner is likely to need more sleep than other people, and it will be sound sleep. Because sleep is so important, so regenerative, its loss or interruption should not be tolerated. Although requirement varies from person to person, that requirement, and the regularity with which it is obtained, should be given priority. Total relaxation is needed if an exercised body is to restore itself. The purely physical benefits of exercise come *after* the exercise, not during. Sleep and rest provide the context in which the benefits can accrue. There is one true test for judging whether you are getting the right amount of sleep; that is, do you wake without prompting? If, in order to be up, say at seven o'clock, you go to bed at eleven and need an alarm clock to rouse you, you are not getting enough sleep and should go to bed earlier. Sleeping should be an absolutely natural, animal process, not requiring prompts or arousals. I doubt whether many animals are insomniac! Since rest and reading can precede sleep, the whole process is one of sheer pleasure. Occasional late nights, or late mornings, are a matter of private choice, but any general difficulty in getting proper sleep should be surmounted stubbornly. I know one athlete who claims never to have gone to bed after midnight and, whilst this example is an eccentric one, it is perhaps a good one, as sleep is 'Nature's balm' and 'chief nourisher in life's feast'.

Recuperation and nourishment are the foundations of a successful running programme, so good food is needed as much as long, deep sleep. Appetite will increase with exercise. Regular meal-times and nutritious food, adequate quantity and balanced mixture (not too much cakes and ale) satisfy the runner's needs without fuss. Care in these areas, of food and sleep, will pay a dividend to the person who has invested in regular exercise. There is no need for diet-sheets or calorie paraphernalia. The favourite food of the great professional long-distance runner Arthur Newton was fruit cake.

Weather will create problems, none of them insuperable, at least in Britain. Rarely would the British runner suffer anything more than discomfort outdoors; cold wind, heavy rain, and sleet will sometimes weaken resolve, but these twists and turns of climate should be ignored, because adequate clothing is always on the market and running warms the body sufficiently for temporary cold to be resisted. Running is carried on in the much fiercer climates of Finland and Canada in winter. The runner has to be decisive in these circumstances, drawing on the terms of his contract with himself, knowing that the difficulty presented by weather is demolished as soon as you get a few yards along the road and scorned when you are back in a hot bath. Heat (again unlikely to afflict north Europeans) is a greater difficulty than cold, though the fitness runner is unlikely to do enough running to risk such catastrophes as dehydration. Clearly, avoid running at mid-day if the temperature is high, largely because there is such discomfort *afterwards* unless a cold shower is available. But it is a matter of acclimatisation; a running friend, Ranjit Bhatia, who lives in Delhi, is not averse to loping along in temperatures above 100°F/37°C, whilst British schoolboys wilt when it is 70°F/21°C. As in the cold, the key is to dress intelligently and not to force training if there is extra strain being imposed by heat. Preferably, wait until the cool of the evening and have the pure pleasure of the late sun.

Generally, as with the actual amount and intensity of running, be alert to your reactions to illness, injury, need for sleep and food, and effect of weather. Judge for yourself in every circumstance, by listening to your physical signals.

The internal, mental difficulties are inevitable and should be cheerfully met and boldly dismissed. They come mostly under the labels 'apathy' and 'disappointment'. You cannot expect always to feel that you want to change clothes and go out to run. Numerous domestic, social, cultural persuasions still work against the regular exerciser, even in the improved background of recent years. But the carrots are there in front of us. The act of running, the sense of movement, the reward gradually accruing in terms of fitness, the possession of something positive, the appeal to imagination; all of these factors, when they are allowed to seep into your mind and life will be persuasive. Pride comes into the situation too. There is no satisfaction to be had from reneging, least of all when you are your own victim. 'Apathy' (by definition, a lack of feeling) is a dreary, uninviting quality. Katherine Hepburn remarked that what she finds intoxicating is the person who says, 'You can do it. It is possible,' and that we live in a civilisation which spends too much of its time saying, 'Well, I don't think so. I haven't got the time.' Miss Hepburn observed that that is a bad way to live and that she likes to identify with something that is on the way up, not with something that is tumbling. Apathy is useless. To say so, will not cure the condition, but to examine and understand the truth of that statement might help to plant a few seeds of action.

Disappointment will be increased by apathy. If apathy rules, nothing will be done; and if nothing is done, there will be disappointment. Disappointment first stems from an apparent lack of progress, but just as progress will be very slow, so it must come. Twenty years of toffees and ice-cream and smoking cannot be wiped out in a few weeks. You overcome disappointment by understanding the true nature of what you are trying to do, which is to reconstruct your machine by strengthening muscles, removing fat, enhancing respiration, neutralising fatigue, and storing energy. This operation cannot be carried out between one Monday and the next. It is not carried out at all by flinching.

It is worthwhile remembering that some athletes (the marathoner, Ron Hill, for example) and all true artists have gone, literally, for years without missing one day's training. At the level of the fitness runner, with fewer demands and less ambition, there really is no difficulty. It has to be accepted, too, that just as any problem of apathy and withdrawal is private and internal, so finally is the solution. Help may be forthcoming from clubs, associations or coaches, but as they say at the end of the old-time music hall evening, 'chiefly yourselves'.

Small practical difficulties are bound to arise domestically at all times of the year. Darkness in winter, the coinciding needs and interests of other members of a family, going away on holiday, slotting the running in with daily demands, each sets a small problem. By careful review before the day, each can be overcome. For example, needing only a half-hour plus time to change clothes and wash, it is always possible to keep going whilst away on holiday, and the alternate-day routine fits easily in the special circumstances, because there is likely to be plenty of opportunity to walk, swim, play numerous games, and thereby supplement the regular running. Fitness can even be proved at this time of the year. Chapter 5 has indicated some of the dodges used by athletes to fit in their training sessions. It is never beyond the wit of man or woman to devise a method or find an occasion, by varying the time of day when you run, by keeping an eye open for places to run and places where you can change, by getting other people to help and maybe join in, by using one or two lunch-breaks, or by watching less television.

It does seem that we have built with our intellects and our technology a society that is deeply contemptuous of our innate physical condition and bodily needs. The car is supreme. The television may be switched on, or over (or off?) from an arm-chair. Even farmers ride around their fields, foresters fell with motor saws, and golfers have buggies. Allied to the work-a-day routine, particularly of the commuter, and to the predominantly commercial, time-consuming tilt of our societies (with all the accompanying good that brings), this technology is subtly antagonistic to health. So long as this is the way we live, and until a happy compromise has been struck, the difficulties of surviving physically and of being active without being eccentric can only be overcome by the knowledge that there is no fun in being sick. The most unfit man is a dead one. There are clear signs, for example in the USA and Britain, that the runner may find himself eventually at the centre of his culture, not out on the edge. As more and more people discover the joy of exercise and the rewards, so the difficulty for those already running, cycling, walking, playing squash, and so on, lessens. The encouraging fact is that this minority is confident, does 'run for fun', and is not likely to be put off, anyway. Stopping would penalise; continuing rewards the doer and might convert the onlooker.

The effects of stopping exercise are soon felt. The regular runner who is forced, by injury for example, to stop will soon feel 'sooted up'. The person who reaches middle-age, having stopped exercise perhaps twenty years before, is in considerable danger from a heart that may not be able to take any strain; he will also have to live with a body that is below par for anything other than the most static physical routine.

Reluctance to exercise can be overcome, therefore, by imagining the rewards of exercise. The act of running, because it is constructive and purely physical, is a pleasure; the result of running is a high level of physical fitness; the places in which the runner moves are themselves contexts for the enjoyment of freedom; and running is a stimulus both to further running and to a more general participation in life, stemming from improved health and increased energy. Once this is experienced and understood, difficulties can be overcome.

9

Some Good Examples

I never take any exercise. I guard against it.
Exercise has done a lot of damage to my
friends.

(Lord Armstrong,
Former Head of the British Civil Service)

Long before Eugene Sandow (1867–1925) advocated a
programme of physical culture and controlled training, there
had been 'pedestrians' who walked or ran huge distances for
wagers. Aristocrats, and the servants of aristocrats, in seven-
teenth- and eighteenth-century England, raced each other,
and competitive athletics was popular in the nineteenth
century, at least as a spectator sport. Even then, age was no
barrier. Sam Mussabini, in his book, *The Complete Athletic
Trainer*, published in 1913, referred to an 'acquaintance'
aged seventy who could run the 100 yards in 14 seconds. Now,
the late twentieth century has brought a recognisable movement, particularly in Western countries, involving tens of
thousands of people in 'jogging' and fitness running. In the
United States, thousands have taken to running (14,300 entered
the 1982 New York marathon), whilst there are 'fun runs'
regularly in most European countries (one in Paris, sponsored
by the newspaper *Le Figaro* drew 30,000 participants during
two days). The USA has a National Joggers Association. The
British *Sunday Times* organised its first national 'fun run' in
Hyde Park, London in October, 1978. Montreal's main park

has road signs barring cars and permitting runners. There are national and international track and field championships for the over-forties. A seventy-one-year-old American woman is said to have completed a marathon in 3 hours 08 minutes.

From a welter of fine examples, I would like to pick a few individuals and a few groups. Their attitudes and their approaches merit attention.

In Anoka, Minnesota, lives Dr William Andberg, who was born in June 1911 and who set an age-group record of 4 minutes 53·2 seconds for the 1500 metres in 1971 and still ran inside five minutes in 1976. (Anyone who does not appreciate this physical feat should take a stop-watch to the track and try it.) Bill Andberg took up running at the age of fifty-five, after a thirty-five year break, remarking, 'I was too fat, getting lazy, didn't feel just right.' Within a year he completed a marathon and at fifty-seven he ran 2 hours 51 minutes for the distance. He acquired a taste for racing, finding that the desire to win was a strong incentive. At sixty-three, he took up ski-racing and in 1978 finished a 36-mile course. Running, he says, is a 'positive addiction' and 'the best thing that ever happened to me'. His maximum weekly mileage in his sixty-seventh year was 70 and during one weekend in May 1978, he raced distances of 3, 6 and 17 miles. Dr Andberg is a runner, not a jogger: 'I run ten miles a day. I didn't say jog. I said run. Arms high, long stride. I never jog. Jogging is hard on the joints. You come down on them, instead of smoothing out.' And his advice on training is direct: 'Listen to your body and train accordingly.' His training route takes him regularly through the Anoka cemetery, and he observed, 'When I'm running over it, I know I'm not under it.' There could be no clearer example of 'positive addiction' than Bill Andberg – or of the remarkable fitness of mind and body that goes with this kind of running, even at such an age.

Amongst a pile of other examples could be found Jack Stevens, running 1500 metres in 4 minutes 50·6 seconds at the age of sixty-five; Noel Johnson, of San Diego, who started at seventy, could jog three miles six months later and then built this to 20–35 miles a week; Fred Grace who completed a marathon in 3 hours 45 minutes at seventy-two; Collister

Wheeler, at eighty-three the oldest competitor in the 1976 USA 'masters' championships; and Duncan Maclean, a Scot who took part in several track meetings when past the age of ninety.

At the other end of the age-scale, fourteen year-old Kathy Miller won the Victoria Sporting Club award in 1978 for sheer courage and example. Kathy was ten weeks in a coma, after a car crash, and later resumed her running.

Between these extremes, there are men and women who, in early middle-age, have performed exceptionally and shown how the delicacy and restrictiveness of most people's approach to physical activity could be thrown away. New Zealander, Jack Foster, started running at thirty-two, being able to jog for twenty minutes on alternate days; eight years later, he ran in the Munich Olympics marathon and finished eighth. In 1974 he ran the Commonwealth Games marathon in the extraordinary time of 2 hours 11 minutes, and he again contested the Montreal Olympics marathon in 1976, finishing seventeenth. Foster has noted, 'I am one who believes it is the mind which needs working on most.'

Australian Percy Cerutty, who coached Herb Elliott to his Olympic gold medal, was near to being a physical and nervous wreck at the age of forty-three, so he set about healing himself, going into the Australian Alps and seeking hard physical exercise. In the early days, he could run a slow quarter-mile. Later between the ages of forty-eight and fifty-five, Cerutty ran 4300 miles. He lived into his eighties.

Joss Naylor, a Cumbrian sheep farmer, has completed possibly the most remarkable piece of running for a man of nearly forty. Naylor covered the 271 miles of the Pennine Way, from Kirk Yetholm, Roxburghshire, to Edale, Derbyshire, in 3 days, 4 hours, 36 minutes; he did 106 miles on the first day, 80 on the second, and 68 on the third, over very hilly, rough country. Brian Harney, of Rotherham, has since run the distance in 3 days, 0 hours, 42 minutes, confirming what kind of stress can be withstood.

These extraordinary examples show what can be done. Few people will follow to such limits, but at least the rest of us will know how far out those limits are and be aware that our own barriers are too careful and protective. Also, it is clear that men and women of all ages have enjoyed such accomplishments. Not only is the sense of fitness and well-being worth having for itself; the fact of achievement is satisfying, even when the achievement is very private. Everything points towards the value of this 'positive addiction'.

Also persuasive is the example of someone who finds, too late, the importance of exercise. In 1977, the General Secretary of the British Trades Union Congress, Len Murray, suffered a heart-attack. Mr Murray was later to lend his name to the Health Education Council's propaganda for a 'Fitter Britain', admitting that, before his heart trouble, his daily exercise was little more than 'getting up and walking downstairs'. After the attack, he started to exercise daily and to walk at the weekends – 'I feel a much better and brighter person for it.' It is a pity that physical illness has to be the late motivation for taking exercise, and it is doubtful whether fear of illness or death does motivate many people, but the red light that signals the break-down of the machine is sometimes noted and is flashing regularly. The green light that beckons positively is more to be recommended.

Most people need the encouragement that comes from a group, or perhaps an individual or an organisation. There are running groups scattered throughout most Western countries now and many of these have developed the idea that the group must meet regularly and be something more than a casual coming-together of casual runners. For example, in Staffordshire, the 'Stone Jogging Club' hires a school changing-room and draws as many as a hundred runners to a session; the Club has an annual dinner and awards.

Some enlightened business houses have their own fitness gyms and facilities, just as many organise and support a range of sports teams. In London, Rank Xerox have a gymnasium at their Euston Road HQ and this is open at 7 a.m. and has an established programme. Fitness can be tested and measured, plans designed for individual employees and advice given by a professional. Not many commercial or industrial concerns will go to such lengths, yet the provision of a single bath- or shower-room might be enough to encourage those who would go for a lunch-time run, or travel to work on foot or bike. Initiative is needed and initiative is prompted by concern. Where there is enough imagination to create concern, the rest follows. Everyone benefits from this kind of enterprise.

A feature of wealthy countries, and an example of what can be done to promote running and other forms of exercise, is the local 'sports centre'. In Britain, there are many, on the pattern of the Crystal Palace national 'centre'. Whilst fitness running need not make demands on these buildings, or on their professional personnel, they can serve as meeting places, offering changing accommodation and washing facilities, even road or grass circuits for the runners.

In the summer of 1983, I visited a typical centre, the West Borough Sports Centre, Maidstone. In addition to badminton and squash groups, there was a general 'keep fit' class in the gymnasium, and a fitness-running group. Runners could use either a one-mile parkland circuit or a two-miles road circuit, and these circuits were, of course, open to the keep fit group. When the fitness-running group was first established, a chart, ruled to show each hundred miles achieved, was kept on the wall in the entrance to the building. Throughout the winter, runners met every Monday and the ages of participants ranged from ten to fifty; numbers taking part fell from about forty to a half-dozen when regular persuasion and encouragement was not forthcoming, and the lesson here does seem to be that most people (certainly beginners) need constant cajoling and want to have their activity arranged and pushed, either by a strong-minded person or a core of enthusiasts. This is puzzling, since it is the participant who benefits from his or her efforts and gets the pleasure from the activity. Initiative is always at a premium. Membership of the West Borough Centre, at that time, cost £6.80 for an adult, with an 80 pence charge per session. More than 2000 people belonged.

These individual and group examples show what is involved and what can be done. The barrier of age is seen to be a flimsy one, easily broken by anyone who wants to break it. The limits to physical endeavour are much wider than most people would think and the ground leading to them is exciting and open to anyone who has the spirit to try. The process is enjoyable, because all that is derived from it helps the actor physically and mentally. Exercise is a positive force, worth running into.

10

Clothing and Gear

He was dressed in a flannel shirt, flannel trousers and night cap, lamb's wool stockings and thick-soled leather shoes.

(Description of Captain Barclay Allardyce, given by Walter Thom, in *Pedestrianism*, pub. 1812)

Running kit has changed since Allardyce's day. The shirt would now be a cotton T-shirt, the track-suit trousers would be nylon, tapered or flared and in at least two colours, the night cap is now a woollen hat, the stockings wool and nylon, the thick-soled shoes certainly thick-soled and possibly leather but brightly coloured, adorned with brand strips, and shaped for the space age. It is useful, though, to look through the enormous range of styles and colours, of shoes, vests, suits and accompanying items, in order to find those garments which will allow running to be comfortable, and free of injury.

Starting from the bottom of the body, it is wise to remember that a lot of running must be done on roads and that they are unyielding. A half-hour of road-running will mean that the feet hit this hard surface more than two thousand times each; the totally unnatural ground can do a lot of damage to feet, legs and back, unless something soft is placed between foot and road. That something is the thick sole of a modern, specialist shoe, probably with two layers of rubber/sponge above the sole and below the foot. Here we are encountering another form of stress, directly physical but not particularly welcome or useful.

In comparatively slow fitness running, the runner lands mostly on a flat foot, with weight and pressure directly and substantially on the heel. The cushion of flesh under the heel could be bruised, the muscles and tendons of the whole foot strained, and the larger muscles, tendons and ligaments of the lower and upper legs pulled, with further possible damage to the lower back. An over-weight beginner might do formidable damage in all these areas. This is neither a false alarm nor a reason for withdrawal; it is a plea to the runner to be fussy about shoes.

There are five basic types of running shoe, three of which merit serious consideration by the fitness runner. You could buy a straightforward 'road shoe', coming in dozens of colours, patterns and combinations of material, but essentially with a nylon or leather upper and a synthetic sole; or a shoe with a 'ripple' sole, which is to say one cut deeply like the edge of a saw; or a studded shoe, with moulded studs not unlike those in football boots; or a 'waffle' shoe, which has many very small rubber studs almost completely covering the sole; or spiked shoes, meant for track racing. The waffle and the spiked shoe need not concern the fitness runner, though for different reasons. The very small waffle studs give only a slight grip on slippery surfaces and wear out quickly on hard ones. Spiked shoes are for competitive athletes. A studded shoe will be valuable to the runner who can run regularly in woodland or fields, where the surface yields and grip is needed; they can be obtained with a degree of built-up heel and with uppers made from glossy synthetic material which prevents mud from clinging. The ripple sole helps also in these circumstances but suffers from drawback, which is that it affords no grip when a slope is being traversed (when the studs would still hold). Ripple-soled shoes give better protection under the foot, though, should there be much road mixed with your country. All in all, they are the most practical shoes, if somewhat heavy. But it is the road shoe that must be examined and selected with care. What is said now about selection and fitting of a road shoe applies, of course, in general to any of the other types. This is not a case of being finicky or ostentatious. There really is a lot at stake, if a course of fitness running is to be carried through successfully and enjoyably.

First, go to a specialist runners' shop, not to any local branch of a chain store; there is nothing wrong with a chain store, but it rarely sells the very best sports shoes – and would you buy golf clubs or climbing boots there? Similarly, it is not wise to use mail order firms though specialist runners' shops do supply a lot this way and are sure to understand your needs. Really, shoes which are going to allow your feet to beat the ground thousands of times should be selected, fitted, felt and fussed over, or money may be wasted and choice regretted. The worst that can happen with a running shoe is that there should be a point in the upper which pushes onto the foot; a row of stitches, a ridge, or just a stiff area will cause extreme discomfort. The front of the shoe, particularly, should be pliable, so that the continual roll of the foot, operating force-fully on the rear joints of the toes and on the ball of the foot, does not work against resistance, to raise blisters. And a firm heel is vital, with a cup built into the upper. The idea of a tab, lying close to the heel and to the Achilles tendon, is favoured by some and condemned by others; defendants say that the tab gives protection, opponents that it may damage the tendon. In practice, neither is likely, because the tab is very soft and the pressure is slight. It is useful to grab when putting a shoe on!

Running shoe uppers may be leather, mock-leather, nylon, nylon with added suede support, or completely suede. Leather, if properly cared for is probably superior to all the others, though expensive. Nylon is popular, giving a closer fit than most materials; the problem of over-heating has, to some extent, been overcome by making the upper into a mesh, to allow air through to the foot. Suede tends to stiffen when it has been used in wet and muddy conditions regularly. The vital quality to be looked for in the uppers is, in fact, this one of suppleness, so that nylon will again be favoured. One or two of the most recently developed leather substitutes are worth considering, because they are, and remain, soft.

The key area is the heel of the shoe. Every good running shoe will offer protection there, probably three layers of it. The first layer, contacting the ground, should be tough enough to survive at least a year's pounding by a fitness runner; the second will be a layer of sponge or rubber, where softness is not necessarily a virtue, because of the enormous and direct pressure down through the heel; and the layer which contacts the runner's foot will be added comfort in the form of a 'sock' or 'inner sole'. Each of these three layers should extend to the toes.

Overall, there needs to be perfect comfort, giving the illusion of running on thick grass and adding to the pleasure of the exercise.

I would also mention a 'prayer mat', which is amusing to the uninitiated observer but is practical and hygienic if you are changing in public dressing-rooms. A twelve-inch square of nylon kitchen matting is better to stand on than a cold cement floor, which may harbour the verruca bug.

Socks should be cotton with reinforced nylon soles. Full nylon would last but, added to the nylon upper of a shoe will not allow the feet to breathe, so causing discomfort and possibly blisters. These reinforced socks are thicker than usual and will emphasise the need for careful shoe fitting. Vaseline or talcum powder on the toes will prevent rubbing (vaseline more effectively because it can be smeared on, under and between the toes).

Commonly, runners suffer from the 'athlete's foot' skin irritation. This itching torment can be allayed by 'Mycota' cream or by 'Dr Scholl's' powder and by careful drying between the toes. It may, however, recur and persist.

Whether you go running in shorts or tracksuit is essentially a personal choice. Many older people will be embarrassed if bare-legged in the street, hesitant if bare-legged in the park, and even self-sonscious in the woods. In winter, tracksuit trousers are fine, in summer most uncomfortable and hot. Whether using shorts or trousers, cotton is cooler. Shorts should be running shorts with freedom of movement allowed by the particular cut, especially at the sides.

Amongst vests, there is a choice of singlet (cotton or nylon) or long-sleeved (or T-shirt), depending largely on how cold or warm it is; and over this a tracksuit top or 'sweat-shirt', with or without a hood. Cotton vests are completely superior to nylon, which trap sweat. A string vest is an option well worth considering. The top garment may be fleece-lined cotton for use in winter, but the fitness runner is unlikely to require a hooded top; that garment is for the athlete before a race on a cold day. Over-heating is not an enjoyable feature of running, neither is it a way of reducing weight, except for the few hours until lost liquid is replaced. So, knowing that exercise will create warmth, it is advisable to wear too little rather than too much. There has to be plenty of trial and error – particularly error. Fashions change regularly, and so do attitudes, as is shown by the words of the author of a late nineteenth-century book on athletics, who wrote:

> A word may be said about the practice which some men have recently tried to introduce from America of wearing sleeveless jerseys, which display the whole of the shoulder and the armpit. There is nothing to be urged in favour of the practice. A light sleeve over the shoulder cannot possibly impede a runner any more than a cobweb would, and the appearance of a runner with his shoulders and armpits uncovered is far from picturesque. Happily, when a runner appears so clad, his usual fate is to be marched off the track, and told that he will be allowed to come on again as soon as he is properly dressed, so we are little likely to be troubled with sleeveless jerseys in the future.

But, troubled we are!

On the market, too, are the so-called 'wet suits', overgarments for top and bottom, efficiently resistant to rain and cold wind. If made from material known as 'Gore-Tex', the suits are quite expensive but very successful in allowing body heat to escape, whilst preventing the penetration of water. If made from nylon, they keep out rain and snow, but keep in warmth and remain somewhat cumbersome. Less sophisticated, cheaper top garments are probably adequate, more comfortable, easy to obtain and to renew.

From the heat of summer to the cold of winter, clothes

worn for running may vary from shorts and vest (sleeveless jersey!) to shorts and vest beneath nylon trousers, sweat shirt with or without hood, and possibly a woollen hat and gloves. But, when you reach the stage of being able to run for a full half-hour, there will be little problem keeping warm unless you live where extremes of weather are experienced. Even there, the essential 'core' warmth will soon be generated by continuous running.

One small incidental item which proves useful is the tennis-player's wrist band, a small piece of towelling which helps greatly to keep sweat out of the eyes.

Every other page of an athletics magazine now carries an advertisement for some piece of runner's clothing. Every trick of colour and shape has by now been employed, particularly in the design of shoes. Elements such as thickening and softening the soles, or making the whole item lighter, can be accepted as a contribution to safety and ease of movement. Beyond this, there is a lot of superfluous fashion and change for the sake of change, which can be ignored. Quality, comfort and practicality are the watchwords.

11

Programme, Diary, Check-List and Chart

Let diaries, therefore, be brought into use.

(Francis Bacon)

A programme, in one or two phases according to preference and intention, can then be put into practice. It may also be helpful to record what running is done and check particular elements in the programme.

The first phase of the running programme, sketched at the end of Chapter 6, can now be exemplified in some detail. A second plan is also offered, for those readers who may decide to see how much further they can go. Each half of the programme should be tailored by the individual, to meet his/her needs and circumstances. What is offered here is a plan that would work for the person who is a complete beginner, out of condition, and needing the suggested minimum six-month period of effort; followed by a plan which would lead to a level of fitness somewhere near to that which a competitive athlete might consider sufficient as a base. You can, of course, start at any point in phase one or phase two, according to your known, present fitness; thus, the programme is useable for six months, or a year, or any portion of a year.

Programme, phase one: (sessions at least every other day, and each session lasting about a half-hour)

| Weeks 1 and 2 | walk, relaxed but above strolling pace |
| Week 3 | include 6–8 stretches of 20–30 metres |

running, just lifting enough to feel the extra strain on muscles – use this week to test your running capacity

Week 4

if week 3 was manageable, continue with the short running stretches, to get confidence and remove any soreness – if you were not ready for running, go back and repeat weeks 1 and 2

Weeks 5–8

establish a base of running stretches

Week 9

double the length of each running stretch OR of as many of these as you can (overall distance now being run is about 400–500 metres)

Week 10

if week 9 was manageable, continue and establish the longer running – if not, go back to weeks 5–8

Weeks 11–16

consolidate the running – keep your movement fluent, relaxed, rhythmic – observe and note your physical reactions, particularly pulse-rate

Week 17

attempt to lengthen all or some of the running stretches

Week 18

consolidate week 17 – running is now about half of your exercise, still in separated sections – this is important for recovery and development

Weeks 19–24

(as for weeks 11–16)

Weeks 25 and 26

link the running stretches (the moment of truth!) at least for the first or last 15 minutes of the session – it is important to take the first 5 minutes or so at a very easy pace, to loosen off

| Week 27 | either consolidate the half-hour run or go back to week 24 and build again until able to enter week 25 |

When you arrive at the end of phase one, consider the value of building on the foundation you have now laid. If you decide to go on, pursue the following programme.

Programme, phase two: (sessions at least every other day and each session lasting about a half-hour)

Week 1	insert a 'fartlek' session on one day, lasting the full half-hour – maintain the regular running on other days
Weeks 2 and 3	repeat the single 'fartlek' once each week
Week 4	include a session (*instead of* the 'fartlek') on a track or on firm grass-land, running a series of 100 metres at a speed greater than anything you have yet attempted, but not yet at full strain – walk to recover after each, then run very easily for about 15 minutes to finish
Weeks 5–10	get one session of either 'fartlek' or 100 metres each week, maintaining all other running sessions regularly (every day, if you can)
Weeks 11–20	try to include a long session at the the weekend, either running easily for up to an hour or doing an hour's 'fartlek'
Weeks 20–26	piece together the whole training pattern you have so far tackled, of steady running plus the faster sessions of varying kinds – maybe, attempt a heavy track session of stretches longer than 100 metres

Finally, about a year after starting, run your original half-hour course and time the effort. This will be both a serious piece of running and a boost to morale, because the run will take less than thirty minutes! Incorporate this occasional timed run into your overall plan.

By now, after about a year, you will be fitter than you thought possible. Further progress lies entirely in the imagination and can be achieved systematically by gradual increase of pace in all sections of the established sessions. Improvement will breed improvement; function will determine structure. The enjoyable 'fartlek' sessions can be lengthened and extra fast stretches included. Track sessions can contain more, and faster, stretches. Sustained runs can be faster. The challenge is always there, the game becomes more and more enjoyable, the satisfaction increases with an increase in capacity. At no time need you use more than the original half-hour, though on a summer's evening when you are mixing the pace through woodland you will feel persuaded.

To record your running in a diary is to establish an explicit incentive and reminder. Specialist diaries can be bought, but are too elaborate for the fitness runner's needs. A cheap desk-diary is sufficient and can be adapted quite easily. Such a diary might incorporate a ten-point checklist, articulating all the achievements, and intentions, of the progressing runner. Six of these points will be relevant to every session, whilst the other four provide the means for a general review of your current accomplishment.

The list is:

1. Which course you run on;
2. The type of session done (e.g., how much running in the early stages; or, what kind of set session if you move into phase two);
3. Time taken;
4. Level of fatigue, on the five-point scale, with Fl as slight and F5 as not acceptable or desirable;
5. Pulse-rate, on finishing, at three hours afterwards, and the following morning (it is interesting, too, to note pulse on a day when no running has been done);

6. Amount of sleep and rest;
7. Days achieved, each week, month and year;
8. Progress measured on a (subjective) ten-point range, assessed monthly, with Pl = very slight, P5 = very satisfactory and noticeable, P10 = unlikely except where at least six months elapses between one assessment and the next; and, on an (objective) measurement of the time taken to run a set course, or even to walk/run it;
9. A statement of targets, say for the next month, especially if you have slipped back;
10. Current attitude, honestly assessed and stated, and what affects it.

This diary checklist has no magic in it, but it is a device for keeping clear what you set out to do and to what extent you have done it. The end persuades the means, so the means need to be visibly prompting.

The practical alternative to a diary is a wall-chart, made from graph paper and adjusted to the purposes of the runner. This can be done by using thirty-one squares on a horizontal line against the name of the month written on the left; a second row below this, for the fatigue index; and a third for the pulse-rate. A tick is placed in each square of the first two where on that day a run was accomplished. When there has been a definite and apprehended improvement, a red line is drawn round that square. If you know, and measure, that you have slipped back, draw a black one! Thus, the ladders and the snakes are located and recorded. At the bottom of the sheet, points seven to ten of the checklist can be written up. All of this requires only a very small piece of paper, which could be pasted to the foot of the bed for the absent doctors to be told about.

By these means, running is established, developed, recorded and prompted. The whole enjoyable, profitable process becomes what it should always have been – an essential part of an intelligent routine, paying the best kind of dividends to the shrewd investor. But it happens to be free.

12

Moving On to the Marathon

You do not run 26 miles on good looks and
vitamin pills.

(Frank Shorter,
Olympic marathon gold medallist)

If the two programmes outlined in the previous chapter have
been completed, there arises a major temptation – the marathon.
It is not only fashion and publicity which have given the
marathon its popularity. This distance is stamped with the
authority of time, even if the story drawn from Herodotus does
tell of a run of 160 miles done in two days and the Greek
athletes did not race anything like the 26 miles 385 yards
(42,195 metres) which was the distance of the 1908 London
Olympics marathon and is now the accepted length of all
marathon races. Whatever the original truth, a long run, by
Pheidippides, is associated with the Greek city of Marathon
and a battle fought there in the fifth century BC. The word
and the modern event have caught the imagination of large
numbers of people, issuing a challenge to a small corner of the
urban psyche. Television cameras record the pageant of the
London and New York races and these events are amongst
hundreds now held all over the world. What Emil Zatopek
said – 'If you want a race, run the 100 metres. If you want
an experience, run the marathon' – is being endorsed by tens
of thousands of men and women. But, before biting this apple,
consider the implications.

First, notice that a lot of pretending goes on. Is the marathon to be run, or partly walked? To claim to have *run* a marathon when it takes longer than $4\frac{1}{2}$ hours is to make an essentially false claim. Covering the miles at an average of more than ten minutes each is not running; go onto a track and complete a lap in $2\frac{1}{2}$ minutes for proof of this. That an inexperienced, or old, person should complete 26 miles on his or her legs is totally admirable and to be encouraged, but if it is your intention to *run* a marathon, think in terms of 3 hours 59 minutes as your closing time.

Therefore, admit that this is difficult territory to enter. The two six-month phases should first be accomplished. From this base an attempt may be made, if time can be afforded and if the desire is there. It would be a good idea, first, to discover one of the many measured marathon courses and go round this on foot, walking and jogging perhaps. Any fit person can walk 26 miles, give or take a sore toe or two. It might even take eight hours, but a sense of the distance would then be imprinted. To run this distance, however, is physically and mentally extremely difficult and will require a minimum of 9 to 12 months' deliberate preparation and progress, from the base already explained.

Racing-distances are all arbitrary, none more so than the marathon. Therefore, training has to be pitched somewhat towards a special required effect. A bias of effort and activity is created, against a background of general running and recovery. 'Mileage' is the measure of this bias, showing the extent to which the body is being taught to do the special thing it will eventually be asked to do. A run of some twenty miles will become the aim, to be achieved several seeks before a marathon is attempted, to confirm physical and mental capacity and thus promote confidence – or perhaps to issue a warning and act as a stimulus. In order to get this twenty miles, there will have to be a range of training activity which always centres on sustained running, but which allows and admits other kinds of running, for variety and recovery.

Sessions to be used are: $\frac{1}{2}$ hour and 1 hour sustained running (probably covering between 5 and 9 miles); as the training develops, relaxed runs reaching to 12–15 miles, done once a

fortnight during the fourth to ninth months; fartlek sessions of
1–1½ hours; track/grass sessions of 200 metres at fast-striding
pace, with brief recovery walk/jog. It has to be emphasised
that it is the cumulative effect of many days' running which
matters. Fitness is extended ever so gradually, not with the
sudden wave of a training wand. Amongst these sessions there
must be rest and recovery, according to the individual, current
state of fitness, and to pressures from the rest of life. Thus, for
example, a day when 3 or 4 miles of very easy running is done
might count as a rest/recovery day. The holder of the USA
5000 metres record, Duncan Macdonald, said 'The ability of
my body to do what I ask of it determines what I do each day,
each workout. Rest is as important as stress, form and concentration are as important as strength – and the proper
balance of all these is the ideal I try to obtain.'

With mileage at the centre of preparation, and with the
possibility of anything from six to fourteen runs a week, the
total distance covered in a week could reach 200 miles. It will
not, in practice or intention; though the New Zealand coach,
Arthur Lydiard, did experiment and go to 240 miles in one
week, he found, of course, that such running is both un-
profitable and stale. It is doubtful whether 100 miles will be
needed weekly by the fitness runner wanting to achieve a
marathon. Jack Foster rarely sought even 80. On the other
hand, it is there to be enjoyed, as Ron Hill – who runs thirteen
times a week – pointed out. At the other end, it would be
unwise to think that 26 miles can be run inside four hours by
anyone who has a foundation of much less than, say 40 to 50
miles weekly. Most serious track runners will do more.

So, a two-weeks cycle of the plan will contain six really
strong, sustained efforts of anything up to ten miles; one or two
fartleks; one or two sessions of 200 metres; and as many sup-
portive runs, an easy 3 to 5 miles, as can be slotted in, sometimes twice a day. You begin to feel really good! Chemical
reserves are high, musculature is toned, the running is easy,
wintertime or summertime. The more you do, the more you
want to do. Therefore, as the weeks pass, the sustained efforts,
which are at the core of the running, will more often be above
an hour and the pace will increase as fitness allows it to.

The remaining aim will be to insert a 20-miles run, whenever this is thought to be manageable, after months of regular running. If it can be done, then put another one in, in each two-weeks cycle; mileage will be raised to 50–60 a week. This should do.

Further contribution to the process can be made by entering some road or cross-country events. It is not necessary to be an avid competitor, but there is no final substitute for the sort of edge put on to fitness by being with lots of other runners, many of whom will, logically, be faster than you. Measurement of fitness against the watch, too, will be quite categorical and persuasive; a 10-miles race, for example, will indicate very clearly what stage has been reached in the long haul towards enduring 26, and something around 75 minutes for the 10 miles might be expected, with 80 minutes satisfactory and 90 too slow. It should not be necessary to walk any of the way, because this kind of distance will have been covered already in training, and the several hundred miles by now in the kitty will have insured you. These few intermediate events, aiming a runner towards the final target, should be deliberately selected and spaced. Any club will welcome a newcomer who wants to race cross-country throughout the winter. Such racing will enliven preparation for the marathon, provide good company amongst the fraternity of running buffs and, incidently, strengthen the whole structure of athletics by recruitment. Essentially, there is no incentive as strong as a race, without which the training may sometimes be thought not to matter, even if it is enjoyable. Students tend to take more care when exams are coming up! Not only do the challenge, excitement and apprehension attached to a race have an appeal; there is enormous satisfaction in looking back at one that has been accomplished, at whatever level. In any case, despite the popular fun-run philosophy which now pervades distance-running, the sport is essentially competitive, and even apologists for fun-running talk of 'everyone being a winner' in the competition against himself or herself. Racing provides the circumstances and the challenge.

After as long as eighteen months from the start of the second basic phase (see page 75), you may come to the day of your marathon. As always in tests, especially those which are very demanding, there will be apprehension before and on the day. There is no answer to this, only acceptance and careful readiness. Physical preparation is, by now, done with and tricks learned in training can be enacted and confirmed; light food and drink should be taken as practised, a known time before the start, Vaseline applied to every part of the body that is likely to chafe; clothes checked. It almost goes without saying that the shoes to use are ones which have already been used and are known to be comfortable. Arrive early, so that tension is not increased by last-minute rushing. Even the best athletes have been known to change at the edge of the road just before the race starts and without being able to loosen off. This is not recommended.

The limbering-up process is not crucial for a marathon runner, yet you will always feel better – and slightly less nervous – if you trot for 5 or 10 minutes and stride out two or three times. Other than that, the first few miles will offer the chance to settle into a rhythm, where the body finds its new level of metabolism. As an amateur, you are unlikely to be rushing madly to take the lead.

All that is left now is what Milton called 'new acquist of experience', because there is nothing quite like the race itself and there are always unknown factors which will affect capacity and performance. The extraordinary physical and mental condition required to run 26 miles is not accurately predictable. The race reveals all. Be prepared to empty the reservoir. Take the regular refreshment offered along the way, since dehydration is debilitating and dangerous. Hang on through bad patches, which are commonly suffered but most often survived; other runners will be feeling as bad, or worse. At all times try to judge manageable pace, tuning in to your body. Accept that when deep fatigue is reached, things will be difficult. You will not know you have had enough until you have had enough. There might come a point when muscles refuse. If so, that is no disgrace, and not even as important as it may seem at the time. There is always a second chance, anyway.

If you complete the distance, carry away a small but justifiable piece of pride. Dramatic phrases such as 'the challenge of the marathon' are really very near to the truth, and the challenge will have been met. Rest, or jog briefly, on the next three or four days, according to how you feel, and then plot the next move -- either to go back to a saner routine, enough to maintain a high degree of fitness, or to try again in, say, six months' time. If the latter, it will be enough to re-establish the routine already outlined in this chapter, only this time from deeper foundations, greater speed, better recovery. The *quality* of each training session should be attended to, rather than any idea of increased mileage. Quality means effort and therefore speed. Most people will be happy to fall back a bit. If you are, you should now have enough knowledge of the game fully to enjoy it.

Latecomers to fitness running, especially those who have passed the age of forty, may be encouraged by one or two further examples of the sort of standard that can be achieved. These examples help to dispel fears of what we ought, or ought not, to try. Our physical capacities, though strictly limited, are perhaps too tentatively approached in modern times, which is one reason why we honour those who climb or sail alone.

Jack Foster has already been mentioned, but can well be mentioned again. When he reached the age of 50, he ran the marathon in 2 hours, 20 minutes, 28 seconds, still with the approach of someone who does not let it worry him too much. Just two years older, Dutchman Piet van Alphen competed in the 1983 Rotterdam marathon and recorded 2-22-14. Even further beyond, it is worth noting that Eric Ostbye, at 61, achieved 2-47-46, and that women have food for thought in the 4-10-20 of 75-years-old Mavis Lindgren. As the late Percy Cerutty said (though I am not sure that he managed it), 'Even when they get me in the coffin, I'm going to kick the bloody lid off.' As a motto for marathon aspirants, that will do.

In summary, to run a marathon in under four hours is very difficult, and training will have to be based on plenty of mileage, topped up with some light recovery sessions and occasional fast work, squeezed into shape by racing substantial distance. Strength for the task will be obtained over many months: the event will not be easy. If it is accomplished, the subtle fitness attained might be kept. A sense of achievement certainly will.

13

Some Observations and Ideas

We have not heard the last word on running.

(Alfred Shrubb, 1908)

Age-range for fitness running covers almost the Biblical three score years and ten; at the one end a child will run naturally and inevitably (until told by over-careful parents or the indifferent society not to) whilst at the other, there is ample proof that there is no need to stop until you have to because of physical breakdown. With any luck, that breakdown comes suddenly and completely whilst you are out running! The professional long-distance runner, Arthur Newton, took himself to the end of the road even after he had suffered a stroke. That positive determination accords with a view which was succinctly expressed by an American veteran athlete who said 'People overdo this age crap.'

Athletics clubs always welcome support from fitness runners and membership of your local club would be a practical way of encouraging its growth, helping it to offer athletics to young people, and making your own connection with the sport. A list of all the national governing bodies (who will provide details of clubs) in the English-speaking countries can be obtained from the International Amateur Athletic Federation, 3 Hans Crescent, London SW1X oLN.

Competition may be obtained at all levels and by all ages. Although the majority of fitness runners will not be drawn into competing, the atmosphere and excitement are conveniently tasted at any of the several major track and field meetings held through the summer. Veteran Bill Andberg commented, 'I like the competition and the work that goes into it.' Even if you don't like competition for yourself, you may find that watching others compete increases your interest in running. Major meetings are considerable spectacles, with persuasive atmosphere.

Food should not become a fad. But food is fuel and a body that is exercised regularly needs fuelling substantially and comprehensively. Adequate food will give adequate nourishment; weight is the guide and weight should not vary much, once a high level of fitness has been obtained. Incidentally, whilst a deficiency of vitamins is harmful (as witness the classic connection between vitamin C and scurvy), an excess of them is no help and a normal, regular diet will provide all that is needed. Always allow about three hours to pass between a substantial meal and running, because exercise restricts intestinal movement and the flow of gastric juices.

The *heart* is a muscle and it would seem logical to suggest that, like other muscles, this one is strengthened by use. Elaborate claims are constantly made by 'fitness fanatics', that our most important, life-sustaining organ is given some kind of guarantee by exercise. Such claims are still treated with reserve by many doctors, yet exercise physiologists know that regular running lowers the pulse-rate and increases the stroke-volume. And those of us who run know that we can make heavy demands on our hearts and the demands are answered. Exercise makes the heart work, and function determines structure. It is something more than a guess that indicates a connection between regular, planned running and a strong heart, even if the connection is not an absolute guarantee.

Injury should not trouble a non-competitive runner who grades his/her running effort over many months, allowing strength in muscles to develop. Indeed, injury ought not to strike an athlete; if it does, it is probably a sign of abuse, where too much is done too soon. By wearing the proper shoes, and by not trying to run before you can jog, or jog before you can walk, injury can be avoided. If there is muscle-strain, seek the cause. A careful mixture of walking and jogging, within the limits of discomfort, will normally set matters right. Avoid expensive physiotherapy, because it does for you mostly what you can do for yourself if you go out and exercise lightly. Movement, patience and time are good healers.

Mobility exercises may be of use. Whilst such exercises do little for the fundamental body-metabolism, they do help to free and extend the range of joints, ligaments, tendons and muscles which may be suffering from lack of movement. Mobility exercises need not be elaborate. Common sense dictates that, working down the body, from neck and shoulders to ankles and feet, the joints can be moved, rolled, lifted very simply but quite forcefully. The secret is to put the particular joint through its natural, full range; for example, a knee that has only moved through more than 30° when its owner sits down, should be raised and bent deliberately a few times, and gradually freed. The same, simple extension can be given to shoulders, hips and ankles. Suppleness and flexibility are too often forfeited when they could easily be kept. Running helps mobility, just as mobility exercises help running. Running is, again, much superior to jogging, for the obvious reason that it extends the body's range of movement.

Relaxation is one of the secrets of enjoyable, successful running. To get the most out of running, you have to move fluently, so that the complete cycle of two full strides is free of jerking. This kind of flowing movement, always across the ground rather than up and down on it, also increases mobility in all the joints. Relaxed skilful movement is the hallmark of great athletes and in no way implies lack of effort; effort comes from inside the head.

Salt loss may occur with regular running in summer heat, though the normal daily intake from the normal diet should suffice. 10–12 gm is an average daily amount absorbed and it is unlikely that more will be lost. It is often suggested, though not proved, that there is a link between salt deficiency and muscle cramp, so if muscle cramp is experienced it would be wise to look to salt intake. It is also suggested that there may be a link between salt excess and blood-pressure, so you cannot win them all!

Smoking is a self-destructive process and has little appeal for the runner. To pour hot nicotine and tar onto soft lung tissue is a cynical, unintelligent act and not recommended. A smoker who takes up running is likely to find the early stages very difficult and the lesson a salutary one. With luck, regular and improving running will remove the desire to smoke, so producing a double bonus. Oxygen, by which we live, needs to enter the blood stream through lungs which are clean.

Stitch is a puzzle to exercise physiologists and an annoyance (sometimes a limitation) to runners. The random nature of this particular pain makes it very difficult to identify and explain. Commonly, stitch is said to be a spasm of the diaphragm (the area between stomach and chest), possibly caused by a tugging on the ligaments that connect the large organs to the diaphragm. This pulling may be created by the deeper breathing of the runner, or by his jerky style (often, a stitch comes on in the later stages of a race, or when running downhill), though one leading physiologist noted that the spleen may be involved. Whatever causes the pain, it grips hard and usually forces a runner to stop, which in turn allows the pain to evaporate. Either too much food or none at all will often provoke stitch, graphically described as 'gas in the gut', so the possibilities for prevention or relief are that food should be light and well-digested before a run, that the running action should be fluent, or that a runner afflicted by stitch should relax and walk. Increasing fitness usually means reduced risk of stitch, anyway.

Teeth that have decay in them may release poison into the system and, therefore, affect health. If you are running to keep fit, this is one part of your body which needs regular checking.

Weight-training is a form of exercise which is fairly popular, but which does not mix happily with running. The effect of each kind of exercise is different, and that coming from running is quite superior, especially since it is allied to movement of the whole body and activation of the respiratory/circulatory mechanisms. Weight-training will toughen muscles, tending to shorten and thicken them; running will toughen muscles by putting them through a very full range of movement.

Weight-training is comparatively static and puts strain on heart and lungs by locking the musculature; running is movement and works the heart and lungs in a continuing rhythm of effort and recovery, increasing circulation rather than locking it.